THE BODY SCULPTING BIBLE FOR ABS

MEN'S EDITION

Featuring the 14-Day Ab Sculpting Workouts
The Ultimate Workout Program for the Ultimate Abs

Written by:
James Villepigue

Photography by:
Peter Field Peck

A Healthy Living Book * New York

A Healthy Living Book
Published by Hatherleigh Press
5-22 46th Avenue, Suite 200
Long Island City, NY 11101

www.hatherleighpress.com

Library of Congress Cataloging-in-Publication Data
Available upon request.
ISBN 1-57826-134-1

Disclaimer
Consult your physician before beginning any exercise program. The author and publisher disclaim any liability, personal or professional, resulting from the application or misapplication of any of the information in this publication.

THE BODY SCULPTING BIBLE FOR ABS books are available for bulk purchase, special promotions, and premiums. For information on reselling and special purchase opportunities, please call us at 1-800-528-2550 and ask the the Special Sales Manager.

Cover and interior design by Corin Hirsch

10 9 8 7 6 5 4 3
Printed in Canada

Dedication

Thank you God for giving me the strength, the courage, and the confidence to overcome the dilemmas that we as humans must face in our everyday lives. Thank you for helping me to achieve success and for keeping my faith strong, especially when I needed it most.

I would like to dedicate these books first and foremost to my amazing parents, Jim and Nancy, who happen to be the kindest, coolest, most loving and caring people I have ever had the pleasure of knowing. I love you both and appreciate every bit of love and guidance you have given me.

To my extremely talented sister Deborah. You have come such a long way, Deb. You amaze me!

To my wonderful grandparents, Charles and Gloria, who are the most generous and selfless two people I know. I love you both and want you to know that if you get back even a fraction of the kindness and generosity that you've given to the world, you'll both be blessed with eternal love.

To Stephanie, who happens to be the most dedicated, highly driven and understanding person I know. Thanks for pushing me when I didn't want to budge and letting up when I couldn't. I love you!

And last, but certainly not least, to all of my clients, friends, and family members at the Custom Physiques Fitness Studio in Oyster Bay, New York, and my readers. Thank you so much, for without you, we would not have had this great opportunity to share and pass along this eye-opening knowledge of health and fitness.

—James Villepigue

Special Thanks

Mike Mejia of Spectrum Conditioning Systems (SCS) of Port Washington, New York, provided invaluable assistance in creating this book. Without him—and the use of his facility—*The Body Sculpting Bible for Abs* wouldn't have been possible!

Peter Field Peck's outstanding photography makes our exercises clear and easy to use. Many thanks, Peter.

Jason G., thanks for the being the great friend you are, brother!

Thank you Andrew, Kevin, Lori, Corin, and the team at Hatherleigh, for the fantastic opportunities. Great things to come!

Our models, LoreDana Ferriolo, Mimi Kim, Igor Ladanov, Guillermo Subiela, John Williams (of SCS), and Nana Wolff were troopers during the photo shoot. Thank you!

Precautions

READ THIS SECTION THOROUGHLY BEFORE READING ANY FURTHER!

Always consult a physician before starting any exercise or weight loss program.

If you are unfamiliar with any of the exercises in this book, ask an experienced trainer to instruct you about proper form and execution.

The instructions and advice in this book are not intended as a substitute for medical or other professional counseling.

Custom Physiques, Inc., the editors, and authors disclaim any liability or loss in connection with the use of this system, its programs, and advice herein.

Table of Contents

INTRODUCTION 1
The True Path to Awesome Abs

PART 1: THE SCIENCE OF ABDOMINAL PERFECTION

CHAPTER 1: Know Your Abs 9
Understanding Abdominal Anatomy

CHAPTER 2: Feed Your Abs 15
Proper Nutrition for Extraordinary Abs

PART 2: WORK YOUR ABS

CHAPTER 3: The Warm-Ups 23

CHAPTER 4: Mat Exercises 45

CHAPTER 5: Swiss Ball Exercises 67

CHAPTER 6: Medicine Ball Exercises 93

CHAPTER 7: Equipment Exercises 103

CHAPTER 8: Lower Back Exercises 125

PART 3: THE BODY SCULPTING BIBLE FOR ABS 14-DAY WORKOUTS

CHAPTER 9: The Workouts 141

ABOUT THE AUTHOR 153

RESOURCES 154

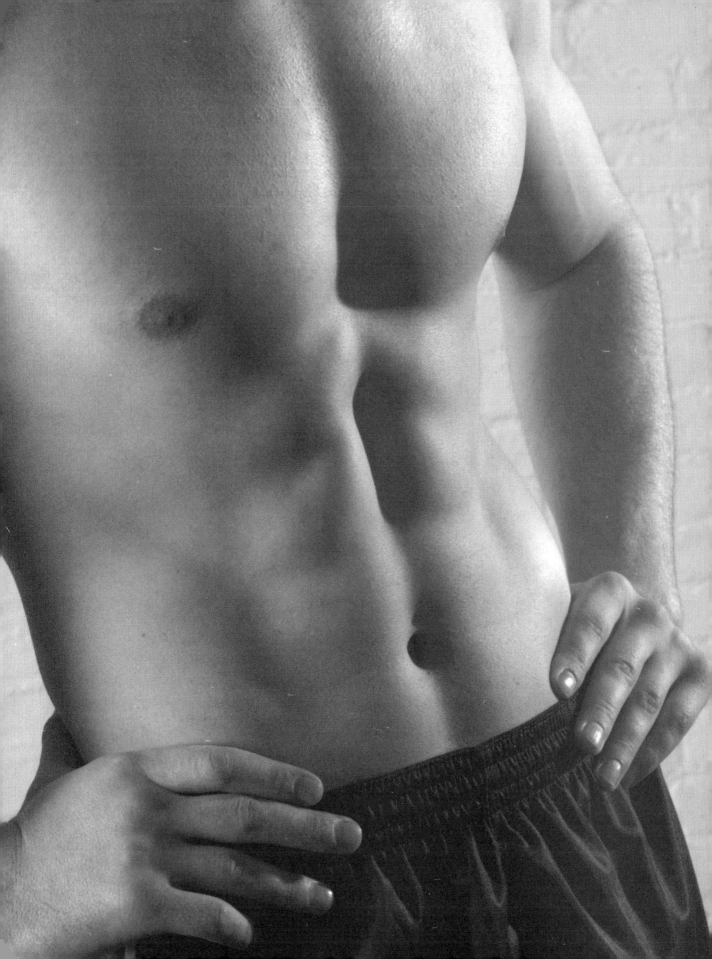

Introduction
THE TRUE PATH TO AWESOME ABS

Forget the starvation diets, the mind-numbing repetitions of abdominal work, and hour after hour spent on the treadmill. We'll help you get the tight, hard-etched abs you've always wanted, but with a much more balanced approach than you've seen in the past. The result? Abs that not only drop jaws at the beach, but also leave your body feeling better and stronger than ever before. So if you're tired of run-of-the-mill ab workouts that don't deliver what they promise, get ready for something radically different!

THE **BODY SCULPTING BIBLE** FOR **ABS**

MEN'S EDITION

A NATIONAL AB-SESSION

So just what is it about the abdominals anyway? I don't mean their obvious appeal; who doesn't want a lean, chiseled midsection? What I can't figure out is why all the confusion. Why is it that almost everyone covets great abs, but so few people are actually able to attain them? Could it be that those chosen few who do sport the elusive six-pack are simply more disciplined than most? Perhaps they have access to some can't-miss workout that miraculously melts away unwanted flab. Or maybe, just maybe, they've been able to filter through all the hype and misinformation about abdominal training and find a strategy that works for them. I'd put my money on the latter.

You see, when it comes to abdominal training there are no ab-solutes (pun intended). What works for one person may not necessarily work for the next. When you consider individual differences in the rate at which our bodies burn fat, varying time commitments to physical training, and different dietary habits, you begin to see why no single approach works best. Sadly though, this simple fact seems to have eluded much of the fitness industry. Cookie-cutter workouts rife with isolation exercises, endless hours of cardiovascu-

lar exercise, and a caloric intake that would barely sustain a hummingbird are too often the recommended prescriptions for a washboard mid-section. And unfortunately, given the relentless manner in which this message has been pounded into the American psyche by both the print and electronic media, it will be difficult to stem that tide.

Much of the problem springs from the fact that in our society a sleek waistline has come to represent fitness and good health. That's ironic, when you consider that appropriately low levels of body fat, while certainly desirable, don't necessarily indicate superior health. Nor for that matter do rippling abdominals indicate a strong, powerful core. And yet many in the mainstream fitness industry continue to perpetuate the notion that attaining a fat-free midriff is akin to reaching some sort of Holy Grail.

Enough is enough! For years now there's been way too much emphasis placed on aesthetics when it comes to abdominal training. The way we see it, what's the point of a washboard midsection if you throw out your back trying to lift a suitcase out of the trunk of your car or picking up a 35-pound toddler. I wish I had a nickel for every time I saw someone with "great abs" struggle to perform simple tasks like balancing on one leg or swinging a tennis racquet properly—never mind those who end up getting hurt because their abdominals and lower back (aka "core musculature") lack the kind of strength they need to perform a given action. How is this possible, you ask? How can something so visually imposing be so structurally unsound? Simple: Performing set after set of crunches and other abdominal isolation exercises, particularly when combined with a lack of lower back training, creates posture and strength imbalances that can lead to possible injury.

THE TOTAL-BODY APPROACH

Here's a shocker: It really doesn't matter how diligent you are about working your abs; if that's all the only training you do you'll never get the kind of development and definition you seek. The metabolic demand simply isn't great enough to make an appreciable change in your body composition. So if you want great abs, you've gotta work your whole body.

THE ISOLATION FASCINATION

To fully appreciate why the traditional approach to abdominal training doesn't work you need to know only one word: *isolation.* And I don't mean working your abs all alone in a dark, dingy basement with nothing but the light of the television to keep you company. By isolation I mean targeting and exercising a specific muscle or muscle group to work without the assistance of others. And when it comes to abdominal training, no exercise accomplishes that task better than the ever-popular crunch. Unlike its cousin, the much-maligned full sit-up, the crunch alleviates undue strain on the neck and lower back and reduces the contribution of the hip flexors. It is this ability to safely and effectively isolate your abs—specifically the *rectus abdominis* (see diagram on page 11)—that has made the crunch the darling of physical therapists, personal trainers, fitness gurus for the past dozen years or so.

The real surprise isn't that this approach failed to produce the desired results; it's that this "isolation fascination," as I like to call it, continues to be so widely accepted. Walk into any gym in this country and I guarantee that you'll see at least a half dozen people mindlessly crunching their hearts out. If they only knew that without necessary dietary modifications and total body workouts that promote fat loss, no amount of abdominal training will miraculously melt away that spare tire. To make things worse, those folks who are working so hard on those crunches are actually promoting postural imbalances that can set them up for future injury.

I'm not knocking crunches; the problem is that people perform them to the exclusion of other ab and back exercises. Look again at the diagram on page 11 and you'll see that the major muscle of the abdominals—the *rectus abdominis*—originates at the breastbone and lowermost ribs and inserts on the pelvis. When it contracts, the muscle flexes the spine to produce an action like the one you do when you perform a crunch. The only problem is that when you do a crunch in the traditional manner—by laying flat on the floor—you're working the *rectus abdominis* muscle through about only half of its range of motion—30 degrees or so.

What it comes down to is that many people do lots of different types of crunches, each kind working the muscle through only about half its range of motion. In the meantime, they virtually ignore the opposing muscle group in the back (it's called the *erector spinae* group, and it acts to extend the spine). What happens? Over time your abdominal wall can shorten and pull your pelvis out of alignment. That places undue strain on your lower back and can wreak havoc with your posture. And for what? Doing all

THE LEAST YOU NEED TO KNOW

• Starvation diets and excessive cardio work can actually slow your metabolism, making it virtually impossible to burn fat.

• It takes a combination of intensive strength training and interval cardio work to provide the foundation upon which great abs are built.

• Constantly working your abs while paying little or no attention to your lower back sets you up for possible injury.

those reps doesn't help you burn any more fat and it doesn't make you stronger because the resistance doesn't provide enough overload. Your muscles can't become stronger if they've already become accustomed to the resistance. You need to push them a little. Why then are so many people convinced that this is the way to great abs? Because that's what we've been trained to believe. Up until now, anyway.

It's time for a fresh start. You want great abs. You need a strong core. This book—with

THE PRE-STRETCH SOLUTION

So the traditional crunch works your abs through only about half their range of motion. The solution, however, is not to sit up a bit farther. Besides being incredibly difficult to do, coming up higher than that 30 degrees taxes the hip flexors to a large extent—not something most folks need to do given the adverse effects that tight, overworked hip flexors can have on proper posture.

The best way to increase the range that your abs have to work through (and the intensity of the resulting contraction), you need to stretch the abs backward about 30 degrees into what I call a pre-stretch position. But bending backward 30 degrees is impossible when you're already lying on the floor. That's where the Swiss ball comes in. Besides increasing the demand on your core musculature to help stabilize your position on the ball, performing crunches on the Swiss ball enables you to drop your head and shoulders back slightly and effectively pre-stretch the abdominals. But what if you don't have a ball you ask? (Don't worry, on page 48 I've described a way you can get this same effect using a common bath towel.)

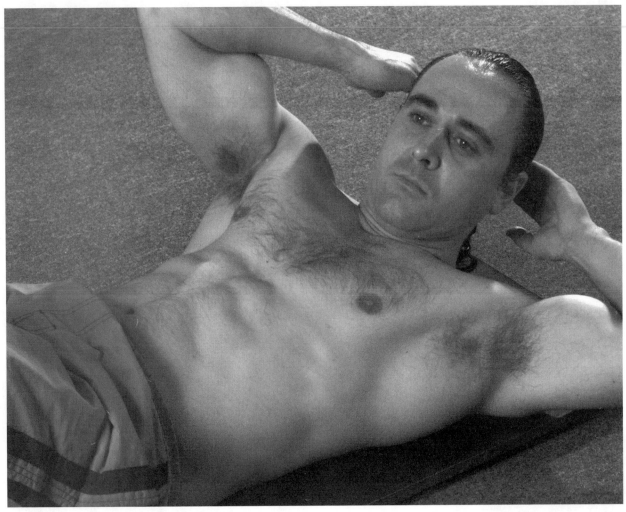

our Body Sculpting Bible for Abs Exercises and 14-Day Workouts—will give you both.

THE 14-DAY WORKOUTS

The 14-Day Ab Sculpting Workout is a system that takes a safe and holistic approach to ab work enabling you to reach your goals in the minimum amount of time. Why 14 days? That's typically the amount of time that it takes most people to get used to a new habit. Also, 14 days is the amount of time that it takes the body to start getting used to a new training scheme. Now, building a habit can be good (waking up early in the morning to work out); but it's not productive for your body to get used to a workout program. Once it does, you'll stop seeing results. (For a full explanation, see *The Body Sculpting Bible for Men*.) And changing your workout every two weeks will keep you from getting bored.

If you've been putting off getting your abs into great shape, now's the time to start. It won't be easy—you have to work for great abs. But I truly believe that this book will get you started. Good luck!

—*James Villepigue*

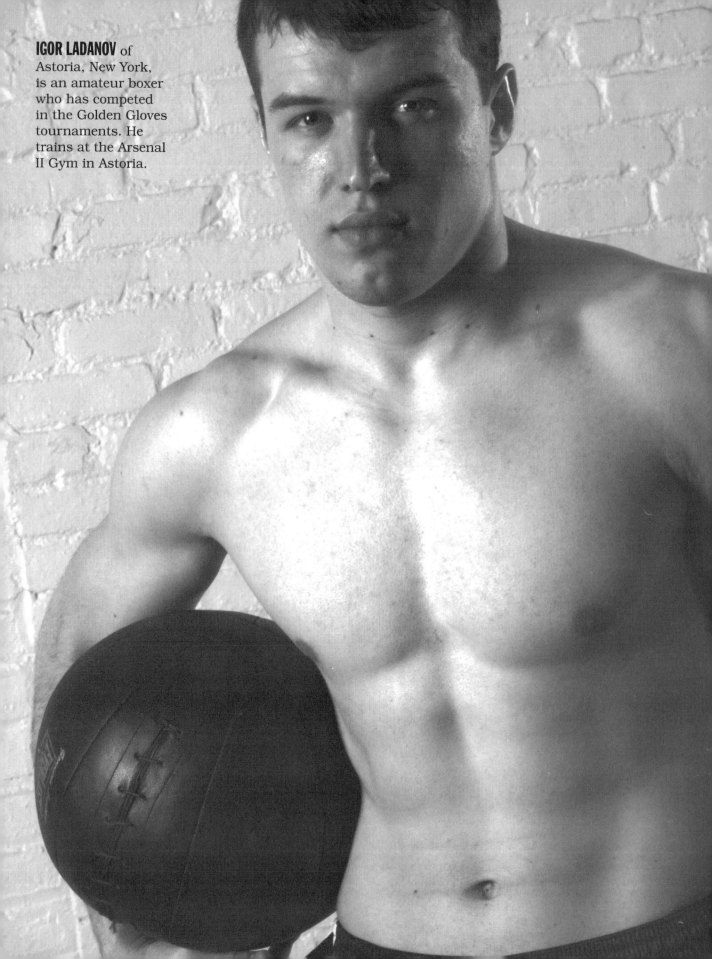

IGOR LADANOV of Astoria, New York, is an amateur boxer who has competed in the Golden Gloves tournaments. He trains at the Arsenal II Gym in Astoria.

Part 1

THE SCIENCE OF ABDOMINAL PERFECTION

Let's cut to the chase. If you want abs—be they sleek, cut, sculpted, or even ripped to shreds—there are three steps you'll have to take:

KNOW YOUR ABS.
FEED YOUR ABS.
WORK YOUR ABS.

Here in Part I we'll explore the first two steps. (Hey—the rest of the book is devoted to Step 3!) In Chapter 1 you'll learn about your ab muscles in a short (I promise) ab-namtomy lesson. After that, you'll find out how to eat right for great abs.

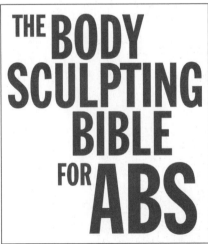

Chapter 1
Know Your Abs:
Understanding Abdominal Anatomy

To achieve abdominal perfection you need to know where your abdominal muscles are and how they work. Here's almost everything you ever wanted to know about the abdominal anatomy—and why traditional approaches to ab training don't work.

1

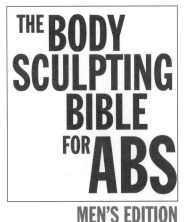

THE **BODY SCULPTING BIBLE** FOR **ABS**
MEN'S EDITION

MEET YOUR ABS

How much do you really know about the structure and function of your abdominal muscles? I'd almost guarantee that you're neglecting at least one of the important ones. This short ab-natomy lesson will help you understand how your abs work—and how you can work them to their full potential.

AB-NATOMY CLASS

To get a better handle on how to train your abs, it's helpful to understand a little about their structure and function. Knowing something about the different parts of the abdominals and how they work is important; when you understand how they work, you'll be better able to train them more effectively. It's been my experience over the years that the more in tune people are with their bodies, the better able they are to push them to perform better. Knowing what muscles you're training and having a mental picture in your mind of how they're moving as they contract during a given exercise helps you form the kind of mind-muscle connection that leads to more focused and productive training. Besides

which, it takes your mind off of counting reps and the gut-busting burn some of these exercises deliver.

The abdominals are made up of a few distinct muscle groups that have a variety of different functions. Take a look at the diagram on page 11 for an illustration of what I'm talking about.

First is the *rectus abdominis*, by far the most well-known of the abdominal muscles. It's what you're talking about when you hear reference to the "six pack." The *rectus abdominis* starts at the sternum and rib cage and inserts on the pubic bone. The primary job of the muscle is to flex the spine, but it also pitches in when you bend to the side (also known as lateral flexion) and trunk rotation. Whenever you do traditional ab exercises, like variations of crunches and leg raises, you're primarily targeting the *rectus*.

The next muscle group is made up of the *external* and *internal obliques*. The external oblique originates on the lateral portion of the ribs and attaches to the crest of the illium; the internal oblique originates on the crest of the illium and fans out to attach to the pubic bone and several ribs. These two muscles work in unison to help you twist and lean.

WHAT'S SO KEY ABOUT THE CORE?

If you do any kind of working out, you've no doubt been hearing the word *core* a lot lately. *Core* is gym jargon for the lower back and abdominal muscles. The core is so important for a number of reasons.

❶ It serves as the link between your upper body and lower body. So, for example, when you swing a tennis racket, you're using your abs and lower back muscles in concert to twist your torso.

❷ The core stabilizes your body during almost any movement: Bending down to pick up your shoes, running to the bus, throwing a Frisbee™, or jumping to reach a blanket from a shelf.

❸ The core protects your body during extreme exertion, like when you're lifting something heavy, whether it's a bag of groceries, an air-conditioner, or a barbell.

MUSCLES OF THE ABDOMEN *(Cutaway view; not to scale)*

The abdominal muscles are arranged in layers. The deepest is the *transverse abdominis* (TVA). It acts like a corset and helps to support the lower back. The next layers are comprised of first the *internal* and then the *external obliques.* They attach to the bottom and sides of the ribs respectively, and assist in twisting and leaning. The *rectus abdominis*, which helps the spine to flex, is one long sheet of muscle that runs from the breastbone to the pubic bone.

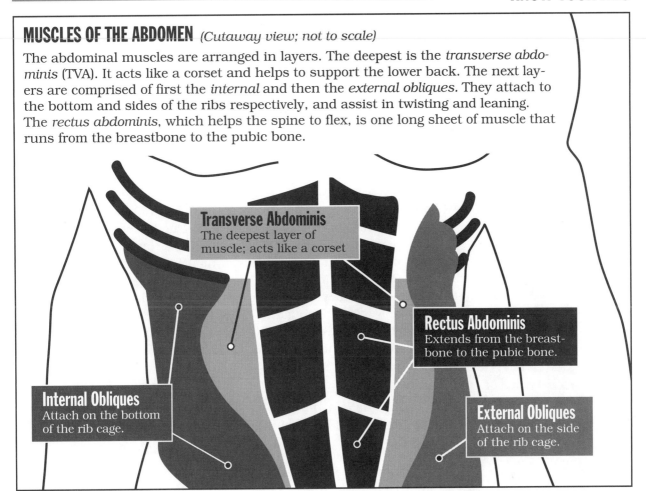

Transverse Abdominis
The deepest layer of muscle; acts like a corset

Rectus Abdominis
Extends from the breast-bone to the pubic bone.

Internal Obliques
Attach on the bottom of the rib cage.

External Obliques
Attach on the side of the rib cage.

The *transverse abdominis* (TVA) lies deep beneath the other abdominal muscles and in fact, most people have no clue that it even exists. That's a shame, because the TVA plays a crucial role in increasing overall spinal stability and is instrumental in proper lifting mechanics. Ever heard a trainer or physical therapist advise someone to keep their stomach pulled in when lifting a heavy object? When you pull in your stomach you're using your TVA to reduce the likelihood of lower back injury. But despite the muscle's vital role in spinal stability, most traditional ab exercises—like the crunch—don't involve it at all.

That's right, cranking out rep after rep of crunches does little, if anything, to train your TVA. So besides running the risk of lower back injury by creating a weak link in your core, not working your TVA can also have adverse effects from an aesthetic standpoint as well. The TVA functions much like a corset by pulling your abdominal wall inward toward your spine. If trained consistently, the TVA can actually help give your waistline a more sleek, hollowed out look. Did you ever notice an individual who had little if any fat on their waist, yet still had a little paunch sticking out over their belt? That could be the result of not specifically targeting the TVA. But don't worry: I've included several great TVA exercises in this book.

HE SAID, SHE SAID

There are some issues about which men and women will almost certainly express dissenting views—the relative merits of channel surfing and the necessity of asking for directions, to name two. So when it comes to working out it should surprise no one that men and women often have different agendas. Given the choice, most guys prefer a buff, chiseled look. Women tend to prefer a sleeker, more "toned" appearance. This holds particularly true with regard to abdominal training. Men typically strive for those deeply etched, bricklike abs and most women prefer a slim, sexy waistline that accentuates their curves.

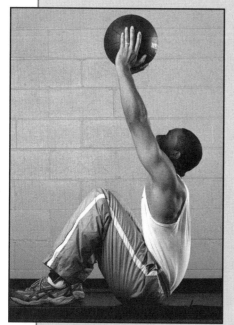

Another way in which men and women tend to differ in their approach to ab work is in their openness to new approaches. Women seem to be interested in trying new exercises; men, on the other hand, will often keep plugging away at the same training routine, sometimes for months on end, despite the fact that they stopped seeing results long ago. Most seem to figure that if they're not progressing they're simply not pushing themselves hard enough, so they just crank up the intensity a few more notches. Ironically, if you guys would just make a few changes from time to time you'd probably see better results with less effort.

So I urge you to try some "new" exercises, like the Slow Sit-Up on page 56 and the Lateral Bridge on page 58. Not only will they improve your ability to lift things without fear of injury, but they will also give your abs a chiseled appearance.

Women may be more adventurous than men about trying new approaches to working out, but when it comes to using added resistance, men take the prize. In fact, men are usually thrilled to add extra weight to any exercise they're doing—whether or not they can handle it. Of course it's a good idea to periodically add resistance to your abdominal exercises because as with any other muscle group, your abdominals need to be progressively overloaded to receive a training effect.

But adding resistance to any exercise, particularly one that involves the abdominals, should be done judiciously. No one's saying that you have to use a ton of weight; just enough so that your abs are fatiguing toward the last few repetitions of the set. Be careful, too, that any additional weight you do use doesn't compromise your ability to do the exercise properly. So for instance, if you're performing a sit-up holding a 12-pound dumbbell over your head and have difficulty completing the range of motion, drop down to 10 pounds. Likewise, if the added weight doesn't provide enough challenge, bump it up a little. The whole idea is to force the muscles you're training to adapt to the new stimulus and become stronger. If you're not doing that you're just spinning your wheels.

COUNT OUT COUNTLESS REPS

Check out the workouts in the back of the book and you'll see that I never ask you to do 50 Slow Sit-Ups or even 25 Swiss Ball Reverse crunches. Here's my stand on high numbers of reps: **They don't work.** In fact, they're counterproductive. Sets of each exercise should consist of 8 to 15 reps (sometimes even fewer). Here's why:

❶ It's the range within which the output of growth hormone is maximized—growth hormone increases muscle and decreases body fat.

❷ Performing that number of reps increases blood flow to the muscles, which provides them with nutrients and helps them recover more quickly.

❸ Keeping the number of reps you do in the 8 to 15 range decreases dramatically the possibility of injury since you need to use a weight that you can control to perform that number of reps.

Now that you know where your ab muscles are and how they work, we can clarify some of the long-standing misconceptions about them. For example: There are no such things as "upper" and "lower" abs. The *rectus abdominis* is one long sheet of muscle that runs from your sternum to your pelvis. When you perform almost any type of sit-up or leg raise the entire rectus abdominis contracts, if for no other reason than to help stabilize your torso. When you perform Hanging Leg Raises (page 114), the lower part of the rectus and your hip flexors do the majority of the work to lift your legs toward your chest; the upper part contracts to help keep you from swinging all over the place. It's true that during some exercises you feel the movement more in one part of your abdominal wall than another, but trust us: The entire muscle is working.

Let's review:

Your abdominals are made up of several muscle groups: the *rectus abdominis,* the *external* and *internal obliques,* and the *transverse abdominis* (TVA).

The oft-ignored TVA muscle can pull in your paunch and help prevent lower back injury—*but only if you train it.*

That's the anatomy lesson. Now as you perform any exercise—whether it's one for your abs, your back, or your biceps—concentrate on the muscle being worked. I guarantee that you'll get better results.

Chapter 2

Feed Your Abs:
Proper Nutrition for Extraordinary Abs

Feeling a little thick around the middle? If there's a layer of fat covering your abs it won't matter how long or how hard you work them. Until you begin to watch your diet and lose some body fat, the rippling abs of your dreams will forever remain a buried treasure.

2

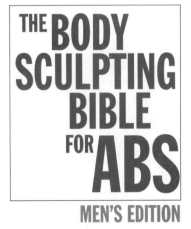

THE BODY SCULPTING BIBLE FOR ABS

MEN'S EDITION

GOOD NUTRITION FOR GREAT ABS

If you want great abs, and I mean really great abs, you're going to need to pay careful attention to your diet. In order for your abs to be visible, many of you will probably have to lower your body fat content. By how much depends on such factors as how high your body fat percentage is when you start and the level of development you want. If all you're looking for is a flat, rock-hard midsection, you won't have to go too crazy with your diet. If however, you want the kind of rippling, chiseled abs that make people gawk when you take your shirt off, you're probably looking at getting your body fat percentage down into the mid to high single digits.

The only way to achieve the kind of eye-popping, head-turning abdominal development so many of us want is to rid yourself of the subcutaneous fat—the fat right under your skin—that otherwise obscures your abs from view. What's the best way to go about this? While there's certainly no shortage of opinions on the matter, finding a method that actually works can be a challenge. Most programs aimed at reducing body fat usually involve drastic caloric restrictions combined with extremely high volumes of car-

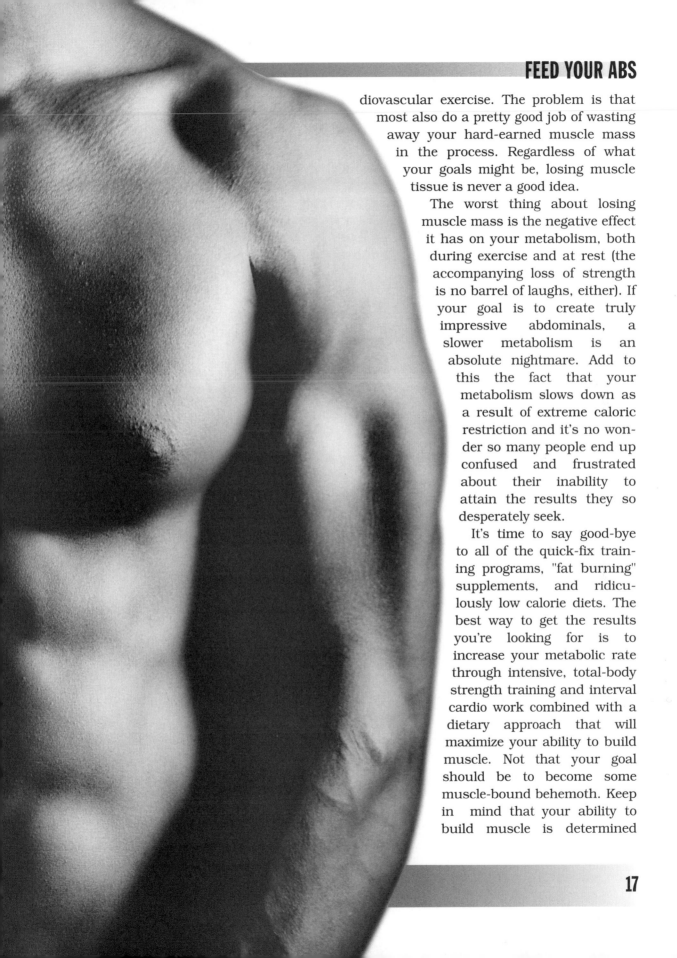

diovascular exercise. The problem is that most also do a pretty good job of wasting away your hard-earned muscle mass in the process. Regardless of what your goals might be, losing muscle tissue is never a good idea.

The worst thing about losing muscle mass is the negative effect it has on your metabolism, both during exercise and at rest (the accompanying loss of strength is no barrel of laughs, either). If your goal is to create truly impressive abdominals, a slower metabolism is an absolute nightmare. Add to this the fact that your metabolism slows down as a result of extreme caloric restriction and it's no wonder so many people end up confused and frustrated about their inability to attain the results they so desperately seek.

It's time to say good-bye to all of the quick-fix training programs, "fat burning" supplements, and ridiculously low calorie diets. The best way to get the results you're looking for is to increase your metabolic rate through intensive, total-body strength training and interval cardio work combined with a dietary approach that will maximize your ability to build muscle. Not that your goal should be to become some muscle-bound behemoth. Keep in mind that your ability to build muscle is determined largely by genetics. However, you do need to eat enough calories to both support muscular gain and keep your metabolism revving at a high level. So how much is enough? It depends on a number of factors including the amount of lean mass you currently have on your body, the rate at which your body breaks down food for energy, and your daily activity level. Check the accompanying sidebar, *Determining Your Daily Caloric Needs* (below) to determine just how much you need to eat.

If your goal is to drop some body fat, use the formula to determine your body's caloric needs and then subtract 500 calories per day from that number. This will be your new daily caloric intake. Even if this turns out to be more (or even way more) calories than you're already consuming, don't worry about it. I need to get your metabolism revving again by getting it out of starvation mode. As long as this increased caloric intake is coming from the right kind of calories (more on that later) and you're doing the kind of total body workouts I outlined in *The Body Sculpting Bible for*

DETERMINING YOUR DAILY CALORIC NEEDS

The first step in determining how many calories you need to consume is to estimate your Basal Metabolic Rate (BMR), which is the number of calories you need to consume each day to maintain basic body function.

BMR = Body Weight in Pounds x 11

A 170-pound man's BMR: 170 x 11 = 1870 calories. That means to maintain his weight, a 170-pound man—even if he sat in a Barcalounger all day—would need to consume 1870 calories a day.

Of course, not many of us spend the day that way. That's why you need to add an "Activity Factor" to your BMR:

Activity Level
Sedentary:	BMR x .30
Moderately Active:	BMR x .50
Very Active:	BMR x .75

Let's say that our 170-pound man is Moderately Active:

1870 x .50 = 935 calories

Once you know your Activity Factor, add it to your BMR, and then add another 10 percent to that total to account for calories consumed by digestion.

Again, using our 170-pound Moderately Active man:

1870 + 935 = 2805

2805 x 1.10 = 3085

He must consume a total of 3805 calories a day *to maintain his current weight.*

A NOT-SO-GRAND OBSESSION

Like any other muscle group, the abs should regularly receive some direct stimulation. In fact, you could argue that because of the crucial role they play in proper posture and virtually all other aspects of human movement that the abs should receive far more attention than muscle groups such as the chest, biceps, or calves.

But—and this is a big but—you should not focus on your abs to the point of obsession, especially if that obsession ends up sabotaging other aspects of your training program. For really great abs (and overall body strength) you'll also need to engage in some form of total-body training and cardio program to help build muscle and boost your metabolic rate.

Men book, you needn't worry about gaining more fat. Making what could be dramatic increases in your caloric intake is going to require you to do much more than just work your abs for 15 minutes three or four times per week.

While it's beyond the scope of this book to lay out an entire dietary plan, the following guidelines should prove extremely beneficial on your road to a lean physique.

Once you've determined your daily caloric needs, divide that amount into five or six smallish meals. This will not only give you a constant influx of protein for building muscle, but it will also help keep your blood sugar levels stable, giving you more sustained energy throughout the day.

I like 35 to 40 percent of my daily calories to come from protein, 35 to 40 percent to come from carbohydrates, and 20 to 30 percent to come from fat. Of course, those percentages will vary from one person to the next.

Consume the bulk of your carbohydrate intake earlier in the day; that's when most people tend to be more active. As the day continues, gradually start tapering your carb intake and upping your protein and fat consumption.

Limit your intake of white flour, white rice, white potatoes, pasta, fruit juices, and other types of "fast acting" carbohydrates. Because they're easy for your body to break down into blood sugar, foods and beverages like these cause a sharp rise in your insulin production to help normalize your blood sugar levels. Besides directing glucose into your muscle cells, high insulin levels also impede your body's ability to burn fat. So, although many of the foods listed above contain no fat per se, consuming them, particularly at times when you'll be less active, can actually increase your chances of storing the calories as body fat. Instead, opt for whole grain breads and cereals, sweet potatoes, brown rice and water whenever possible.

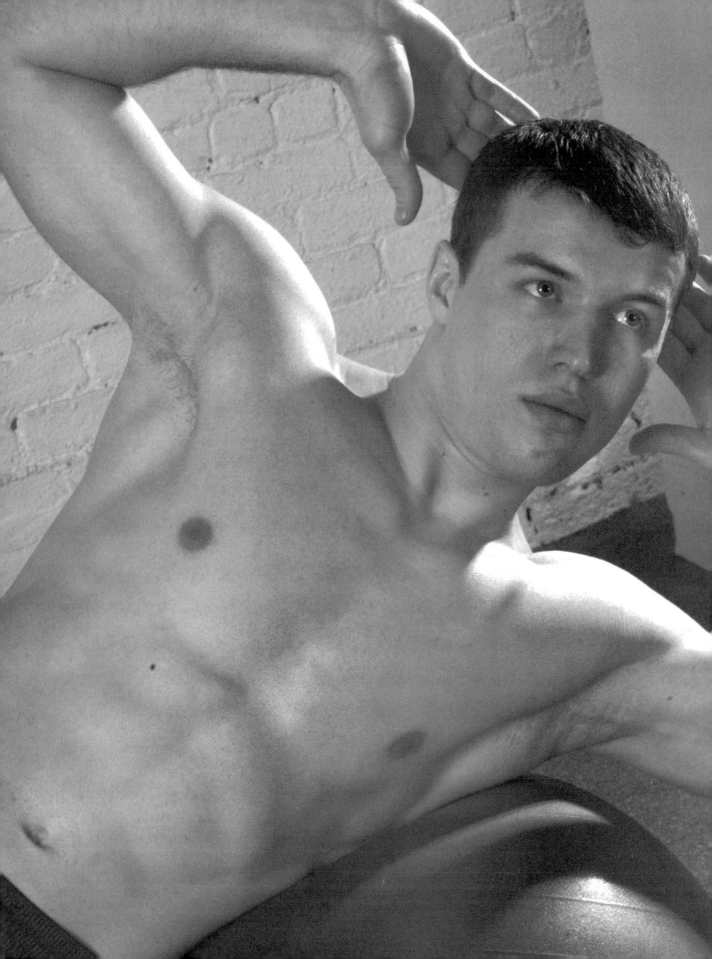

Part 2

WORK YOUR ABS

Here's where we get down to the meat of the matter. From here on out you're going to learn how to do the very best gut-busting exercises available. It starts with an ab-tensive warm-up and proceeds through exercises using mats, medicine balls, Swiss balls, and gym equipment. And by the time you're finished, you'll be the local ab expert.

THE BODY SCULPTING BIBLE FOR ABS

MEN'S EDITION

Chapter 3
The Warm-Ups

Just as you warm up before
you jog or play softball, you
have to warm up warm up
your core before you begin
your abs workout. Here's how
to do it the right way.

3

THE **BODY
SCULPTING
BIBLE
FOR ABS**
MEN'S EDITION

WARMING UP TO YOUR WORKOUT

Before you can get started on your new gut-busting exercises, you need to warm up. One of the easiest ways to injure yourself is to jump into any type of exercise program when your body is "cold." ("Cold" doesn't necessarily mean reduced body temperature, but rather that your body is attempting to go from a resting state into intensive physical activity.) To do that without risking of injury, you need to engage in some form of progressive, large muscle group activity to help raise your core temperature and increase blood flow to your working muscles and connective tissues. This increase in temperature and blood flow helps lubricate your joints and readies them for the kinds of repetitive motions they'll carry out during your workout. It also makes for the easier transmission of nerve impulses that stimulate your muscles to contract.

A general warm-up prepares your entire body for increased physical activity. The most common warm-ups usually involve such activities as running, cycling, rowing, or various forms of calisthenics. Typically these activities are done for a period of 5 to 10 minutes, or until you begin to break a light sweat. This is the way that most people warm-up prior to exercising—or should I say most people who actually bother to take the time to warm-up in the first place.

But as valuable as a general warm-up is, it's not enough to prepare your body for the demands of strenuous training. You also need to perform a specific warm-up to familiarize your muscles and central nervous system with the types of movements they'll be asked to execute during your workout.

By performing some of the same movements that you'll be doing during your actual training session (albeit at a much lower level of intensity), you can bring about more forceful and efficient muscle contractions than you could had you simply knocked out 5 minutes on a treadmill. An example of a specific warm-up would be performing a light set of bench presses with an empty barbell before moving on to more challenging loads. This "wakes up" your central nervous system, allowing it to better synchronize the movement sequence it will experience later under more intense conditions. Think of it as a dress rehearsal; the more familiar your central nervous system is with the exercise beforehand, the more efficiently it can recruit your muscle fibers to contract to produce force.

But how do you perform a specific warm-up for your abs when in many instances you'll be using only your body weight for resistance? All you really need to do is stimulate them with some low intensity contractions that involve such movements as spinal flexion and rotation. Exercises like pelvic tilts, lying on your back and bringing your knees to your chest, and unweighted rotational movements will all help prepare you for the types of exercises in this book. You'll also want to throw in some form of spinal extension and lateral flexion, examples of which I've included. The key is to keep the intensity of these drills low. The idea is to warm these muscles up, not fatigue them to the point where it will compromise your workout performance.

IT'S A STRETCH

After warming up, many people do some form of static stretching for the muscles they're about to train. In static stretching, you bring the muscle or muscles in question into a stretched position and then hold it for anywhere from 30 seconds to two minutes. This is done to relax the muscle and increase its range of motion. The problem with static stretching is

GET YOUR AFFAIRS IN ORDER

Like I've said, besides watching how you eat, you'll need to get your workouts in order. I'm not talking about your ab workouts. What I mean here is the training you do for the rest of your body. To get the lean look you're after, you need to combine regular resistance training with interval cardio work in addition to your ab workouts. There are a couple of ways to do this. Depending on your schedule and individual training goals you can opt to (1) do two or three total-body workouts per week; or (2) choose a more traditional body building split routine in which you train different muscles on different days. Whichever you choose, be sure to incorporate lots of big compound lifts such as squats, dead lifts, bench presses, and rows. For detailed descriptions of how to safely perform these exercises, as well as complete workout routines, check out *The Body Sculpting Bible for Men.*

As for your cardiovascular workouts, the phrase to remember is interval training. Normally when you see someone doing cardio they're usually going about it at a nice steady pace. You very rarely see someone alternating between a minute or so of near all-out work like sprinting and a minute or so of a more relaxed pace, like a jog or a fast walk. That's too bad because that approach will get you fitter, faster and is a more effective way to burn fat. What's that? You always heard that lower intensity cardio work burned more fat? Nope. Working at a lower intensity may burn a greater *percentage* of calories from fat; however, all else being equal, you'll burn more total calories and fat calories by working at the higher intensity. Not to mention the fact that because it's much more metabolically taxing, interval training also offers a much more potent cardiovascular stimulus.

that holding your muscle in the stretched position sends it a signal to relax. That may be fine at the end of a workout, but you don't want your muscles to relax just before your workout, when they will have to contract forcefully. The goal of a post warm-up stretch is to prime your muscles for the increased activity to come, not put them to sleep.

I'm not advocating that you skip stretching before you work out. If you're too tight, you'll have difficulty performing the exercises correctly and increase the chance of injury. The trick is to increase your muscles' range of motion and ready them for the strenuous work to come. The best way to do this is through dynamic stretching. Rather than hold the muscle in a stretched position until it begins to relax, in dynamic stretching you quickly, yet smoothly, bring the muscle into a stretched position and then immediately release it. This sequence of stretching and releasing is then repeated several times. The result is that the muscle "opens up" a bit more each time you stretch it. Dynamic stretching is a far more effective method for preparing a muscle group for the specific demands of the workout and has often been linked to improved athletic performance.

Look at the warm-ups on the following pages and choose three or four to do each time you train your abs. If you train them at the end of your regular strength workouts, these exercises on their own should serve as adequate preparation. But if you give your abs priority by either training them before or on a separate day from your strength workouts, be sure and engage in a five to 10 minute general warm-up period prior to beginning these drills.

Alternating Knees to Chest

This is one of my favorite full-body warm-ups. It is especially effective for loosening and stretching your upper and lower back in addition to getting your abs ready for a workout.

TECHNIQUE AND FORM

1 Lie on your back on an exercise mat with your arms at your sides and your legs stretched straight out in front of you.

2 Bend one knee, pull it into your chest, and then hug it around the shins.

3 Hold this position for one second and then immediately release it back to the starting position as you simultaneously repeat the same sequence with the opposite leg.

4 Continue until you've performed 6 to 10 reps with each leg.

TRAINER'S TIPS

Especially when you're warming up, it is important not to force your joints beyond their range of motion. It might be tempting to squeeze your leg too tightly, but don't force it.

As you pull your knees to your chest, press your lower back into the ground and gently pull your belly button in toward your spine.

If you have tight knees, you can hug your legs under your lower legs, around your thighs.

If your lower back feels tight, go back to your general overall warm-up to increase blood flow to the area.

Alternating Knees to Chest

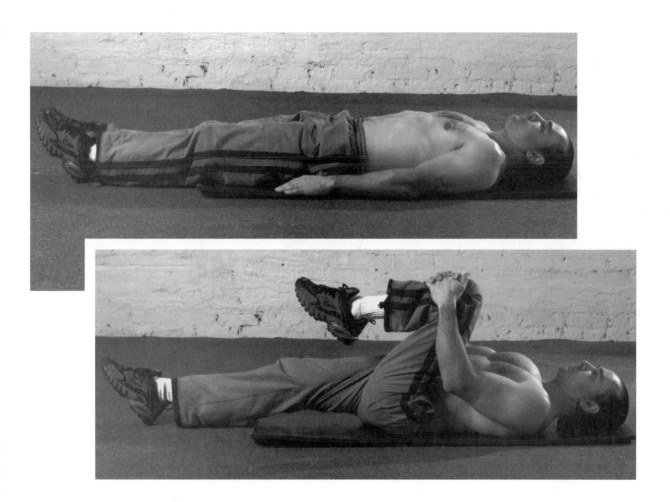

The Roll

Not only is this exercise especially helpful for your upper and lower back, but it effectively targets the TVA, too.

TECHNIQUE AND FORM

1 Sit on an exercise mat with your feet flat on the floor, your knees bent and together, and your chest as close to your thighs as you can get it.

2 Now tuck yourself into a ball: Keeping your heels as close to your rear end as possible, hug your arms around your upper shins and grab hold of one of your wrists. Pull your abdominals in tight to your spine and tuck your chin to your chest.

3 Exhale as you gently roll back until your shoulder blades make contact with the floor.

4 Inhale as you roll back up, contracting your abs and returning to the starting position.

5 Repeat for 8 to 10 reps.

TRAINER'S TIPS

◈ Some people tend to hold their breath during an exercise, but it's important to keep breathing. Pay attention to the rhythm of your breaths as you do these warm-ups.

◈ As with the previous exercise, if your back or knees feel tight, return to a general warm-up before continuing to the exercises.

◈ Make sure to keep your chin tucked into your chest when you roll back.

The Roll

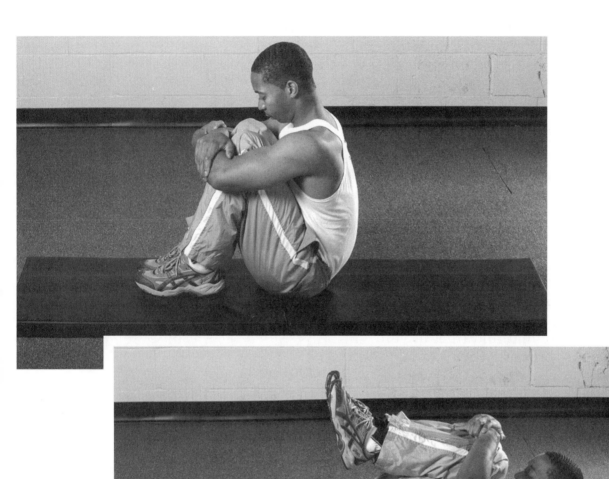

Pelvic Tilt

This exercise will help you find and maintain your "neutral spine"—a position in which your back is stable and less prone to injury. The Pelvic Tilt also gently moves the spine and stretches the lower back. The movement is subtle—but effective.

TECHNIQUE AND FORM

1 Lie on your back with your feet flat on the floor and your knees bent at a 90-degree angle. In this starting position you should have a very slight arch in your lower back, but no more than you would if you were standing up.

2 Inhale deeply and then exhale as you pull your belly button in to your spine. Flatten your lower back into the exercise mat and tuck in your buttocks, pressing them toward the ceiling.

3 Stay in that position for five to 10 seconds and then repeat.

4 Repeat for 10 to 12 reps.

TRAINER'S TIPS

Think of your pelvis as a bowl of water; as you contract your abs and glutes you're attempting to spill the water onto your stomach.

Continue to breathe during the exercise and remember to keep your lower back pressed into floor throughout.

This exercise can also be performed by itself to alleviate sore back muscles.

Pelvic Tilt

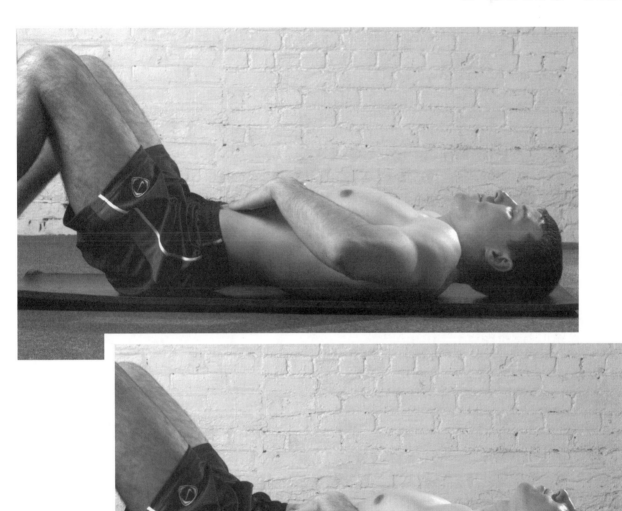

Press Up

This is the classic ab stretch and warm-up. It is sometimes called the Cobra. When you perform the Press Up, remember that in the topmost position you need to keep your hips on the floor and not to lock your arms.

TECHNIQUE AND FORM

1 Lie flat on your stomach with your legs straight out behind you and your hands flat on the mat and next to your shoulders, as if you were going to do a push-up.

2 Slowly lift your torso by extending your arms until your chest and abdominals are off of the floor. Open your chest. In the top position your arms should be straight but not locked.

3 Hold the position for a moment and then repeat.

4 Repeat for 8 to 10 reps.

TRAINER'S TIPS

When you're in the topmost position, your pelvis should still be in contact with the floor.

Never force this stretch; come up only as far as is comfortable—both for your abs and your back muscles.

Keep your lower back and buttocks relaxed during this stretch.

If at any point during this warm-up you experience pain in your lower back, stop the exercise immediately.

If you're not flexible enough to extend your arms for this stretch, you can modify the exercise by supporting yourself on your bent elbows.

Press Up

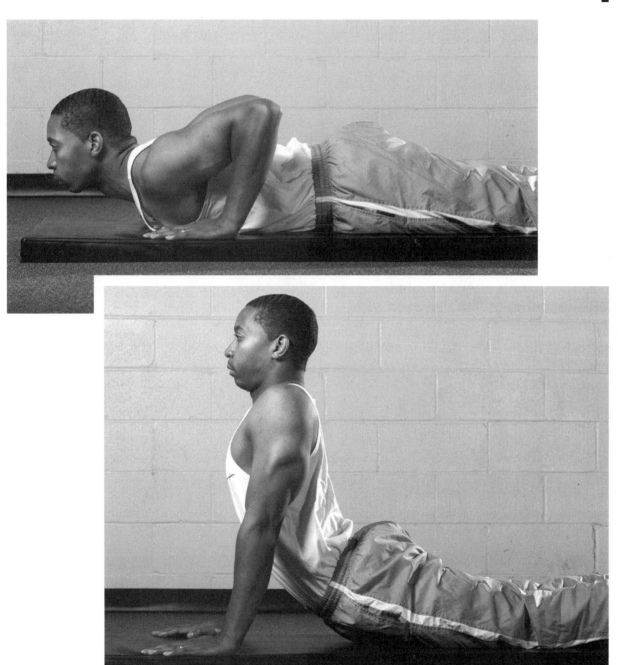

Rotational Stretch

The Rotational Stretch is a great warm-up for your buttocks, hips, and lower back. As with the other exercises, it's important not to force the movement in your hips. It takes time for those muscles to loosen.

TECHNIQUE AND FORM

1 Lie on your back with your knees bent and your feet flat on the floor.

2 With your arms held by your sides, lift and bend your left leg and place the outside of your left ankle against the outside of your right knee.

3 Keeping both shoulder blades completely in contact with the ground at all times, allow the weight of your left leg to pull your right leg over toward the floor.

4 Get as close to the floor as you can before bringing your legs back to the starting position and repeating on the other side.

5 Repeat for 6 to 8 reps on each side.

TRAINER'S TIPS

✪ Remember to keep your upper back and shoulders in contact with the floor at all times during this exercise.

✪ You can vary this warm-up by interlacing your fingers gently behind your head rather than holding your arms by your side.

Rotational Stretch

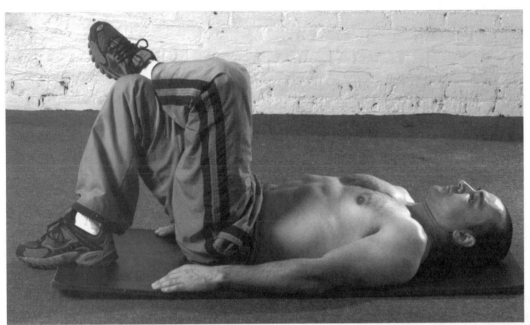

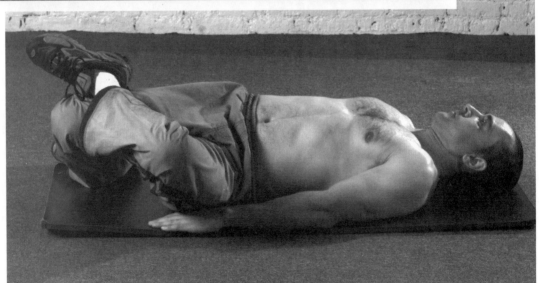

Lateral Lean

In addition to warming up and stretching your obliques and arms, this exercise feels great after you've been sitting all day.

TECHNIQUE AND FORM

❶ Sit at the end of a chair or exercise bench with your legs about shoulder's width apart and your feet flat on the floor. Sit up as straight as possible and extend both of your arms straight over your head.

❷ Slowly flex to one side as far as you can without rotating your torso. Focus on bringing your armpit down toward your hip on the side you're leaning to.

❸ Once you've gone as far as you can (you should feel a gentle stretch on the opposite side), slowly reverse direction.

❹ Repeat for 6 to 8 reps on each side.

TRAINER'S TIPS

✪ This exercise is also effective when performed on a Swiss ball, which challenges your stability and balance.

✪ It's important to keep your torso facing forward during the lean; don't allow it to twist.

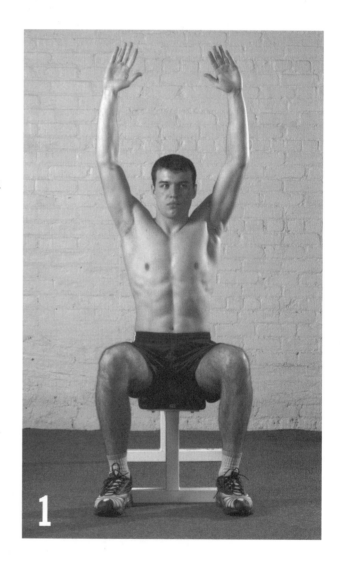

Lateral Lean

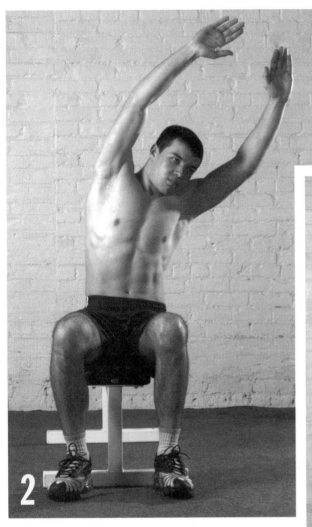

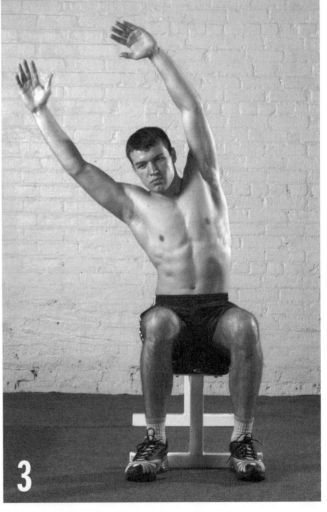

The Angry Cat

Despite its fearsome name, the Angry Cat stretch is terrific for maintaining and restoring range of motion in the back. It also encourages proper posture.

TECHNIQUE AND FORM

1 Get down on your hands and knees on the exercise mat. Position your hands directly below your shoulders and your knees directly below your hips. Look forward, but keep your neck relaxed.

2 With your back arched slightly, inhale deeply and pull in your abdominal muscles.

3 Exhale and round your back toward the ceiling like an angry cat. When you're in the topmost position your chin should be tucked to your chest and you should be pulling your abs in toward your spine as much as possible.

4 Inhale as you drop your back to the starting position and repeat.

5 Continue for 8 to 10 reps.

TRAINER'S TIPS

❖ If you've been diagnosed with ruptured disc or any other serious back problem, you should not do this warm-up.

❖ In the starting position, your back should be sagging gently toward the floor.

❖ In addition to helping you warm up, this exercise is a terrific TVA conditioner—as long as you keep your abs pulled into your spine.

The Angry Cat

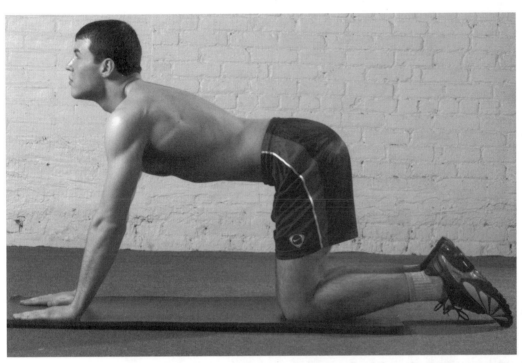

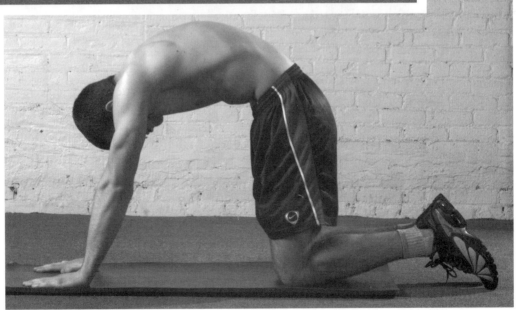

Swiss Ball Pelvic Tilt

Grab a Swiss ball for the next two warm-ups. This one focuses on your TVA and hips. One of the challenges (and benefits) of doing any exercise on a Swiss ball is that you need to balance yourself as you perform the exercise; that builds core stability. This exercise also keeps the pelvic muscles flexible, which helps lessen the chance of experiencing back pain.

TECHNIQUE AND FORM

1 Sit on a Swiss ball with your legs about shoulder width apart and feet flat on the floor. Your legs should be bent at a 90-degree angle.

2 Gently lace your fingers behind your head or place them on your hips or at your sides.

3 Keeping your torso as erect as possible, move the ball slightly forward by pulling your belly button into your spine and rolling your glutes underneath your body.

4 Slowly and smoothly roll the ball back to the starting position and then repeat.

5 Continue for the desired number of reps.

TRAINER'S TIPS

Swiss balls are available in many different sizes. A general rule of thumb is that the ball should be large enough so that when you sit on it, your legs are bent at a 90-degree angle.

During this exercise, your upper body should stay in proper alignment; don't roll or shift with the movement of your lower body.

Swiss Ball Pelvic Tilt

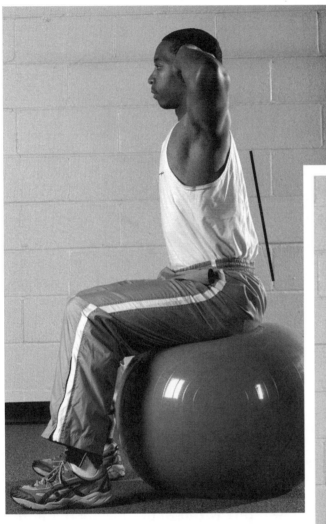

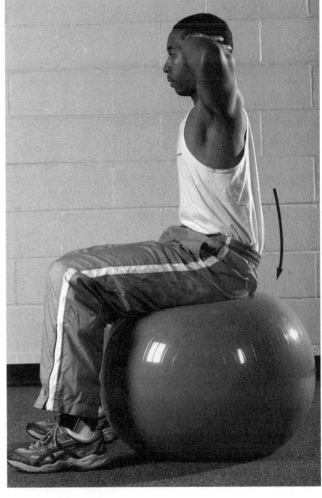

Swiss Ball Figure Eights

As with the Swiss Ball Pelvic Tilts on the previous pages, the Seated Figure Eights help you to maintain flexibility in your pelvis. It also warms up your hips and your legs.

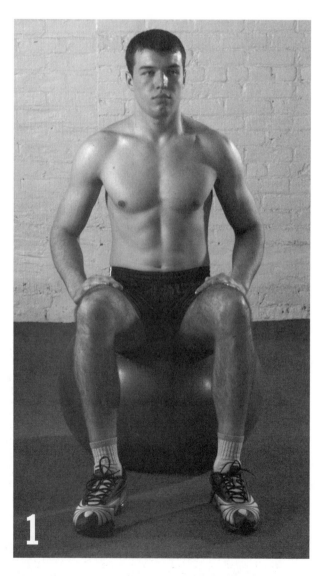

TECHNIQUE AND FORM

❶ Sit on the Swiss ball with your legs about twice your shoulder's width apart and your feet flat on the floor. Your legs should be bent at a 90-degree angle.

❷ Roll your right hip diagonally forward toward your right foot and then very smoothly arc the same hip around and toward your right rear before bringing it back toward your left foot, and then back toward your left rear.

❸ Continue in this figure eight pattern for 5 to 6 reps before changing directions to the other side.

TRAINER'S TIPS

✪ Be sure to do this drill nice and slow; start with small movements and gradually increase your range of motion as you begin to loosen up.

✪ Try not to use your legs too much; imagine that you're tracing a figure eight with your abs and pelvis.

Swiss Ball Figure Eights

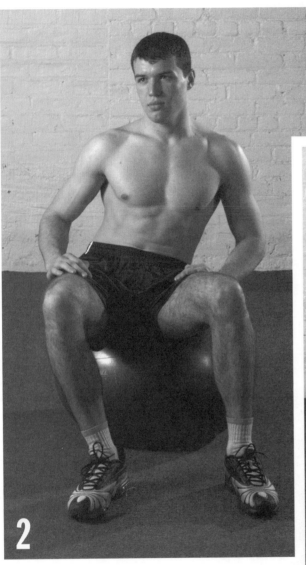

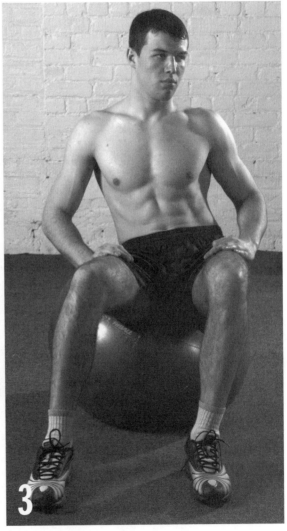

Chapter 4
Mat Exercises

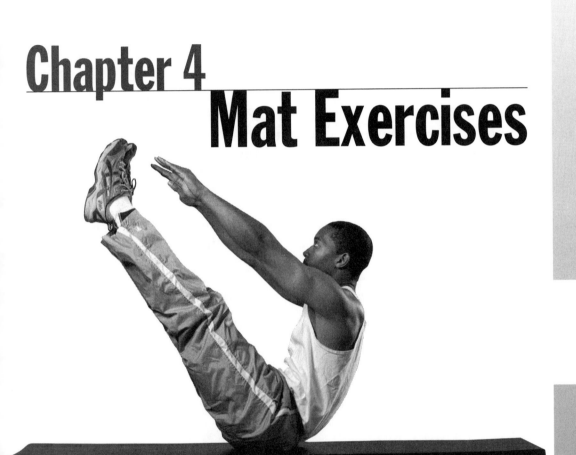

4

There are a number of effective abdominal exercises you can do with nothing more than a simple exercise mat. Sure, it's nice to have access to a bunch of fancy equipment, but as long as you have a mat and are able to perform the types of exercise described in the pages that follow, you can give your abs an awesome workout. In fact, one might go so far as to say that many of the exercise featured here will give your abs a much better workout than they'd get on some of the fanciest gym machines. To get the most out of them though, you'll have to follow our exercise descriptions to a tee.

THE **BODY SCULPTING BIBLE** FOR **ABS**

MEN'S EDITION

Vacuum

Here's a good exercise for targeting the *transverse abdominis* (TVA). To get the full benefit, make sure to concentrate on blowing all your air out to intensify the contraction.

TECHNIQUE AND FORM

1 Stand comfortably, with your knees bent slightly and your back arched slightly.

2 Inhale as deeply as possible.

3 Exhale, blowing out every last ounce of air. As you do so, round your back by pulling your belly button into your spine and dropping your chin to your chest.

4 Once you've blown out all the air, hold the position and breathe through pursed lips for another 6 to 10 seconds.

5 Inhale, extend your spine, and repeat for the desired number of reps.

TRAINER'S TIPS

You can activate your TVA by pulling your belly button into your spine as you exhale. Simply blowing out your air won't do that.

This exercise can also be done from a kneeling position as well.

Vacuum

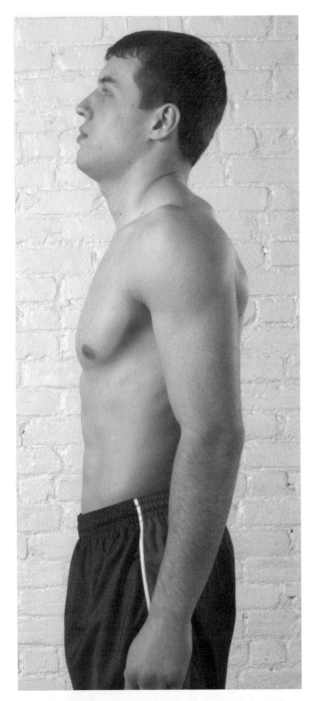 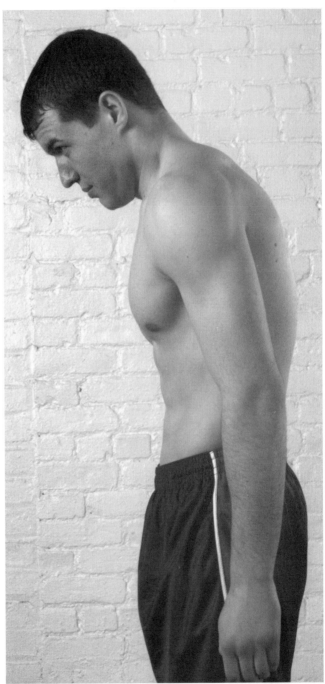

Towel Crunch

By now you know that the traditional crunch doesn't work the abs through their full range of motion. The Towel Crunch helps eliminate that problem by placing the abs in a pre-stretch position, thus allowing them to contract more forcefully.

TECHNIQUE AND FORM

❶ Fold a medium-size bath towel in half lengthwise, and then roll it into a tube.

❷ Lie on the floor with your knees bent and your feet flat on the floor. Place the rolled towel beneath you, just above the small of your back.

❸ With your hands held lightly behind your head, exhale and lift your shoulder blades off the floor by crunching your rib cage toward your pelvis.

❹ When your shoulder blades and upper back are a couple of inches off the floor, pause momentarily before *slowly* lowering yourself back to the starting position.

❺ Repeat for the desired number of reps.

TRAINER'S TIPS

✪ Concentrate on pulling your abdominals toward your spine throughout the movement. This will activate the *transverse abdominis* (TVA) and protect your lower back, especially in the prestretch position.

✪ Make sure your hands are only lightly supporting your head. Clasping your hands tightly and tugging on your head to pull yourself up takes focus off of your abs and places unnecessary strain on your neck.

✪ Exhaling as you execute the crunch further activates the TVA and produces a more forceful contraction.

Towel Crunch

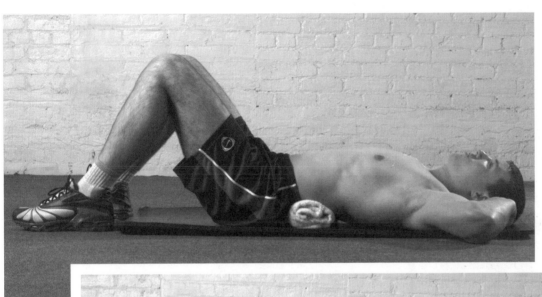

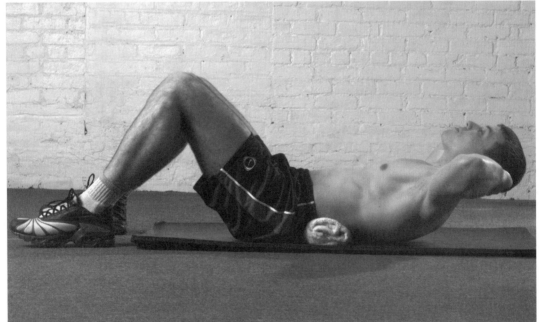

Crunch with Lateral Flexion

This exercise keeps your entire abdominal wall under constant tension while giving your obliques a pretty good workout.

TECHNIQUE AND FORM

1 Lie flat on the mat with your knees bent and feet flat on the floor.

2 With your hands held lightly behind your head, lift yourself into a crunch position.

3 Holding your torso a couple of inches off the floor, bring your left armpit down toward your left hip.

4 Once you've gone as far as you can, hold the position and squeeze your right oblique before slowly returning to the starting position and executing the same movement toward your right side.

5 Repeat for the desired number of reps.

TRAINER'S TIPS

✪ The key is to this exercise is to keep the movement completely lateral. Avoid crunching your opposite arm across your body.

✪ Be sure that you don't allow your torso to lower as you bend laterally. Keep your shoulder blades a couple of inches off the floor throughout the entire exercise.

Crunch with Lateral Flexion

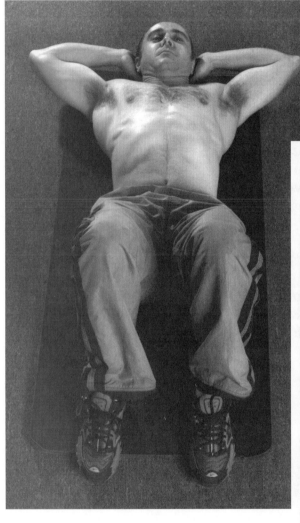

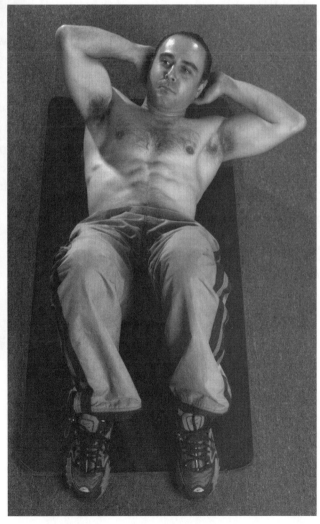

V-Up

This is a very difficult exercise. In fact, the vast majority of people I work with have to work up to it. So take your time, and don't attempt the V-Up until you're ready.

TECHNIQUE AND FORM

1 Lie on your back on the exercise mat with your arms extended straight out behind you and your legs extended straight out in front of you.

2 Pulling your abdominals toward your spine, quickly and simultaneously lift your torso—not just your neck—and your arms off of the mat until your body forms a V.

3 Hold that position for a moment or two before lowering back to the starting position.

4 Repeat the exercise for the desired number of reps.

TRAINER'S TIPS

◆ Although you need to perform the lifting phase of this exercise quickly, avoid using that momentum to heave your legs and upper body off the ground. Concentrate on using your abs to generate the necessary power.

◆ Try to coordinate the movement as best as you can. Lifting one body segment more than or before the other will make it even more difficult to perform the exercise.

V-Up

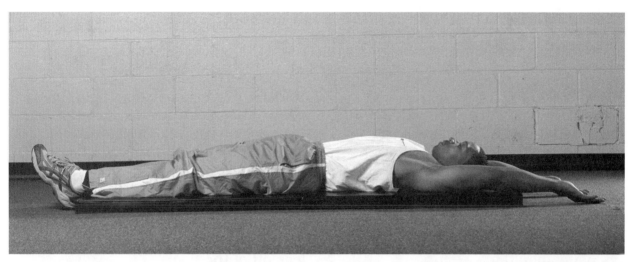

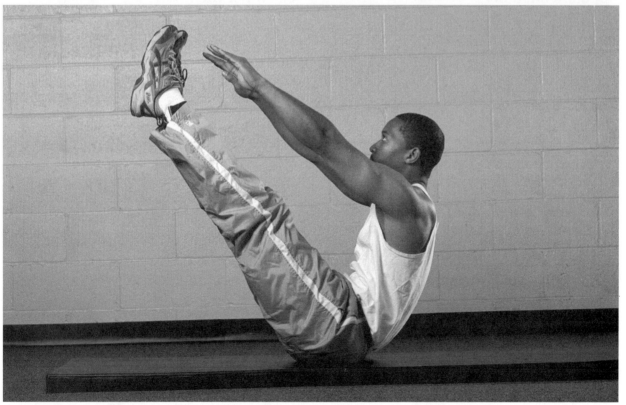

Oblique V-Up

The Oblique V-Up is tough. The trick to performing it correctly is to avoid using momentum to lift your legs of the mat.

TECHNIQUE AND FORM

1 Lie down on your right side on an exercise mat; bend your knees slightly. Your shoulders, hips, and knees should be stacked directly on top of each other.

2 Cross your arms in front of your body so that each hand touches the opposite shoulder.

3 Keeping your right upper arm and shoulder in contact with the mat, lift your legs off the ground while simultaneously bringing your left shoulder down toward your left hip.

4 When you're in the topmost position, your legs should be completely off the ground and your weight resting on your right hip, elbow, and rib cage.

5 Lower yourself back to the starting position and repeat for the desired number of reps before performing the exercise on the left side.

TRAINER'S TIPS

◈ Be sure to keep your feet and legs together as you lift them off the ground during each repetition.

◈ Avoid using momentum to throw up your legs. Concentrate on using your obliques to (1) crunch your rib cage toward your hip; and (2) lift your legs off of the floor.

Oblique V-Up

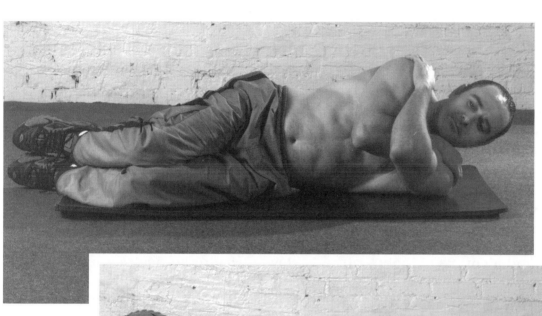

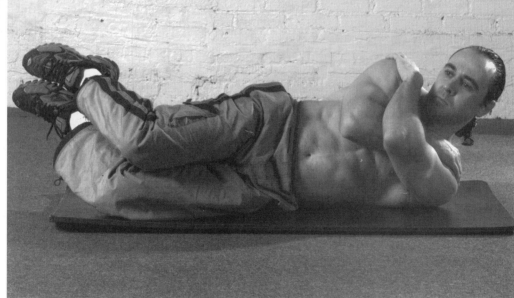

Slow Sit-Up

Despite the fact that they've been all but outlawed by many trainers and rehabilitation professionals, the sit-up remains a safe and effective exercise *as long as you follow two pieces of advice*:

First, do not anchor your feet under anything (such as a barbell or sofa); and second, don't use momentum to throw yourself up off the floor.

By not anchoring your feet, you (1) dramatically reduce the involvement of your hip flexors; (2) make your abs work much harder; and (3) reduce your chances of neck and lower back injury.

TECHNIQUE AND FORM

1 Lie flat on your back with your knees bent and feet flat on the floor. Hold your arms straight and down by your sides and a couple of inches off of the mat.

2 Pull your torso toward your thighs, one vertebra at a time.

3 Once your chest is practically touching your thighs, reverse directions and slowly lower yourself back to the starting position.

4 Repeat for the desired number of reps.

TRAINER'S TIPS

✪ This exercise is designed to increase your abdominal strength, so be sure to sit up and lower yourself slowly. Having to use momentum to get your body going is an indication of an abdominal weakness that needs to be corrected.

✪ If you're unable to lift yourself with your knees bent at a 90-degree angle, move your feet away from you slightly until you're able to properly execute the movement.

✪ The contribution of the *transverse abdominis* (TVA) here is immense. If you don't pull your belly button toward your spine you will not be able to come up.

✪ Keep your feet flat on the mat throughout the exercise.

Slow Sit-Up

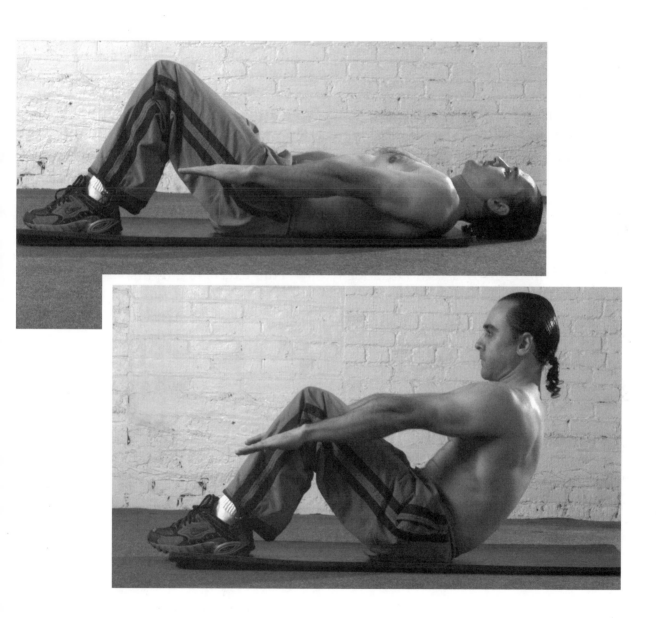

Lateral Bridge

Don't be fooled: The Lateral Bridge may look easy, but it's yet another great exercise, designed to increase your abdominal strength and stability.

TECHNIQUE AND FORM

1 Begin by lying on your right side on the exercise mat. Your shoulders, hips, and knees should be stacked directly over each other.

2 Place your right forearm on the ground, perpendicular to your torso.

3 Pulling your belly button into your spine, push your right forearm into the floor as you lift your torso and legs off the mat.

4 In the topmost position you should be resting on the lateral portion of your right foot and your right forearm, with your right oblique in line with the rest of your torso.

5 Lower yourself back to the starting position.

6 Repeat for the desired number of reps before switching sides.

TRAINER'S TIPS

✪ Avoid using momentum to throw your hips up into the air; that will decrease the training effect of the exercise.

✪ Be sure that the rib cage of the working side doesn't sag toward the floor; keep the bottom oblique tucked up tight into the body.

✪ This exercise can also be done statically: Get into the finish position and hold it for 30 to 60 seconds.

Lateral Bridge

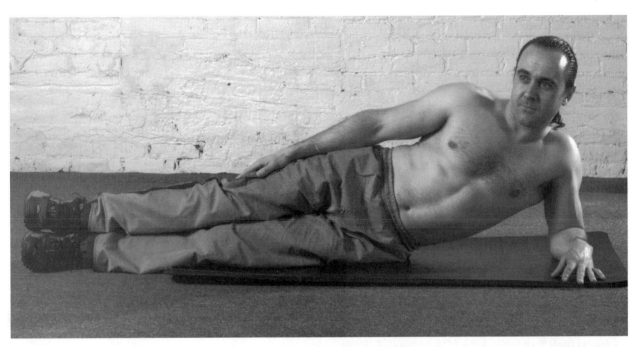

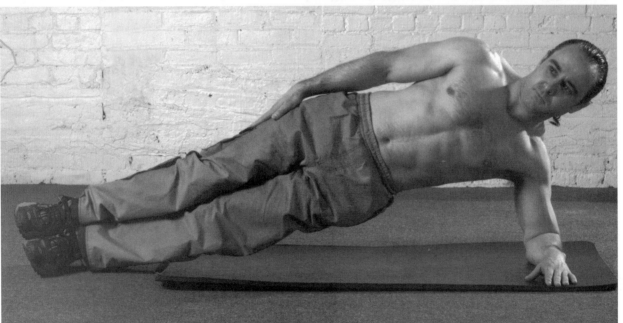

Knee-In

This is another advanced exercise that you may have to work up to. Also, if you have a history of lower back problems, take special care.

TECHNIQUE AND FORM

1 Sit on the mat with your legs stretched out in front of you. Place your arms at your sides with your palms on the mat.

2 Lean backward to the point at which you feel your abdominals working to hold you in the position.

3 Once you're there, draw your thighs toward your chest while simultaneously drawing your chest toward your thighs (keep a slight bend in your knees as you do this).

4 Once you reach the point at which your thighs and chest are practically touching, pause momentarily before returning to the starting position.

5 Repeat for the desired number of reps.

TRAINER'S TIPS

◆ Exhale as you bring your chest and thighs together to intensify the contraction.

◆ Keeping your arms out to your sides will help with balance. For a more challenging exercise, keep your arms overhead as you perform the exercise.

Knee-In

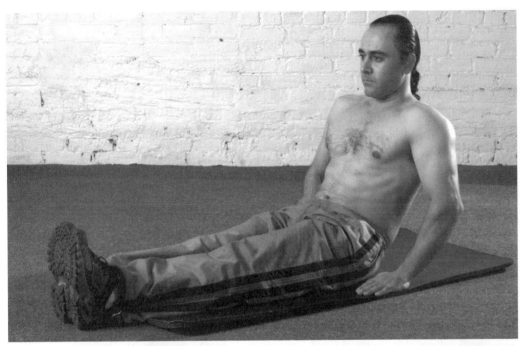

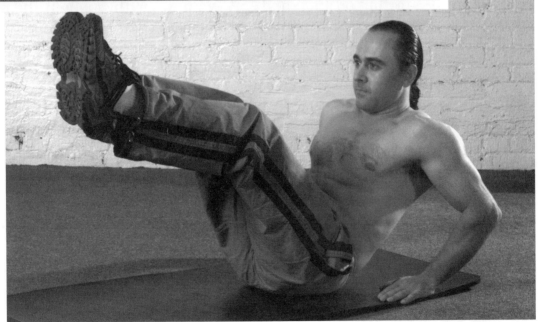

Windshield Wipers

These are great for increasing your rotational strength, although I admit that there are probably better ways to get rain off your windshield!

TECHNIQUE AND FORM

1 Lie on your back with your arms extended to your sides. Extend your legs over your hips with your feet together and soles of your feet pointing toward the ceiling.

2 Keeping your abs pulled into your spine, slowly lower your legs to one side and toward the floor.

3 Get your legs as close to the floor as your flexibility allows before using your abs and obliques to pull them back up to the starting position and then over to the other side.

4 Repeat for the desired number of reps.

TRAINER'S TIPS

⊗ Keep the opposite shoulder blade in contact with the ground as you lower your legs to either side. Allowing your shoulder blade to come off the ground reduces the effectiveness of the exercise and can cause lower back strain.

⊗ Avoid using bouncing at the transition point of each repetition to generate movement in the opposite direction.

⊗ Keep your belly button pulled into your spine throughout the movement. Allowing your lower back to arch excessively can result in injury.

⊗ For a slightly easier version of the same exercise, repeat the movement with your knees bent at a 90-degree angle.

Windshield Wipers

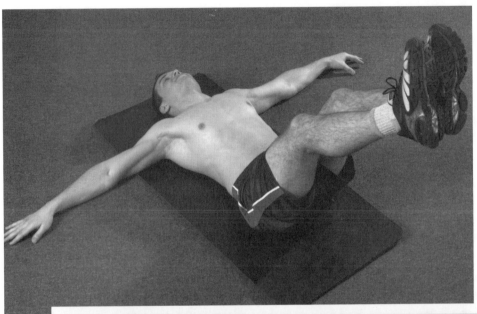

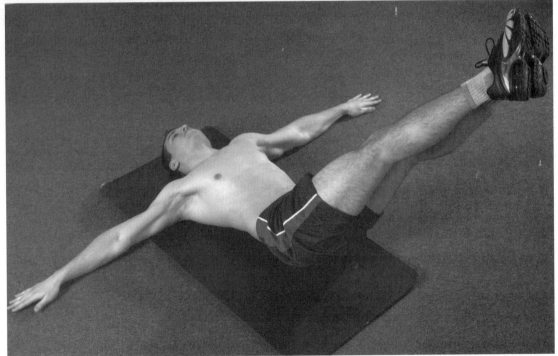

Twisting Pulse-Up

The range of motion may be small, but the abdominal contraction is intense —so beginners beware.

TECHNIQUE AND FORM

1 Lie on your back on the exercise mat with your legs extended toward the ceiling and over your hips.

2 Place your hands, palms down, by your sides or under your tailbone.

3 Keeping your legs as straight as you can, slowly lift your lower body a couple of inches off the mat by pulling your belly button toward your spine and contracting your abs.

4 At the same time, try to twist your lower body slightly by contracting your obliques and pulling your right hip up toward your right armpit.

5 Return to the starting position and repeat for the desired number of reps.

TRAINER'S TIPS

Avoid pushing off with your hands to get your lower body moving up off of the floor. Concentrate on using your abdominals.

Try not to move your legs back toward your head; keep them lifted straight up over your hips.

Initiate the obliques twist by pulling your hips toward your armpit. Avoid spinning only your feet at the top of the movement.

Lift and lower yourself in a slow, controlled manner. If you aren't able, it's an indication that you need to work up to this one.

Twisting Pulse-Up

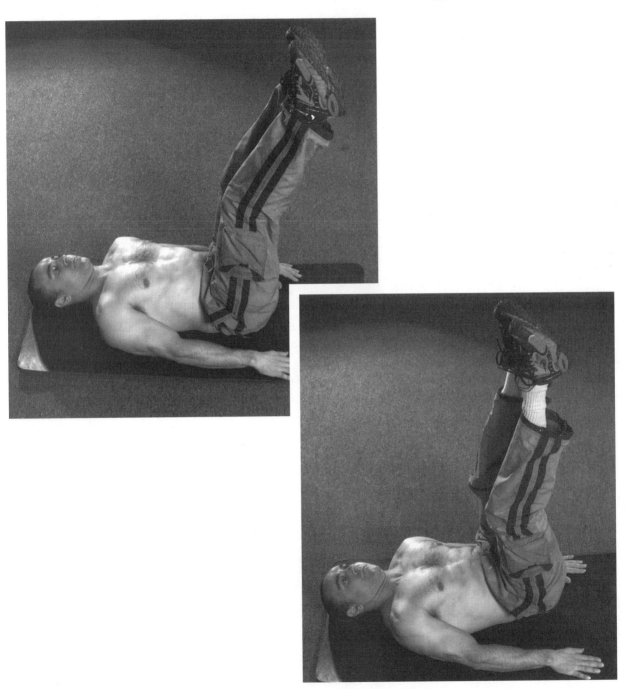

Chapter 5
Swiss Ball Exercises

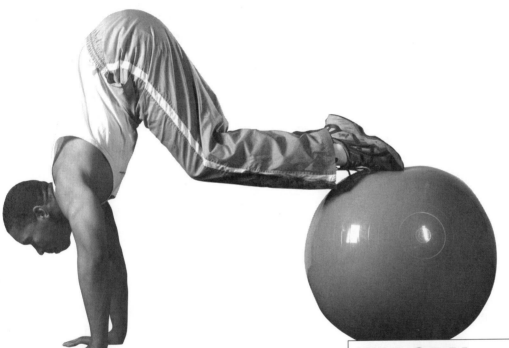

I like to think of the Swiss ball as a wolf in sheep's clothing. Sure, it looks harmless—hey, it's even cute. But Swiss balls are actually one of the most effective and intense abdominal training tools to come around in years. Besides allowing you to work through a full range of motion, the Swiss ball requires you to recruit more stabilizer muscles, thus making any exercise performed on one far more demanding.

5

THE BODY SCULPTING BIBLE FOR ABS

MEN'S EDITION

Swiss Ball Crunch

The great thing about working with the Swiss ball is that it's unsteady. Yes, that's a good thing because it means your abs are forced to work much harder than usual to steady your position. The ball also allows you to work through a more complete range of motion by placing the abs in a pre-stretch position to start the movement.

TECHNIQUE AND FORM

❶ Lie back on a Swiss ball with your hands held lightly behind your head. Your back should be conforming to the ball and your legs should be bent at a 90-degree angle. Keep your hips slightly lower than your torso.

❷ Use your abs to lift your upper back a couple of inches off the ball as you crunch your rib cage toward your pelvis.

❸ Contract your abdominals and hold the position momentarily before lowering yourself back to the starting position.

❹ Repeat for the desired number of reps.

TRAINER'S TIPS

✪ Avoid pulling on your head and neck to initiate your lift off the ball.

✪ Exhale and pull your abs toward your spine as you execute the crunching motion.

Swiss Ball Crunch

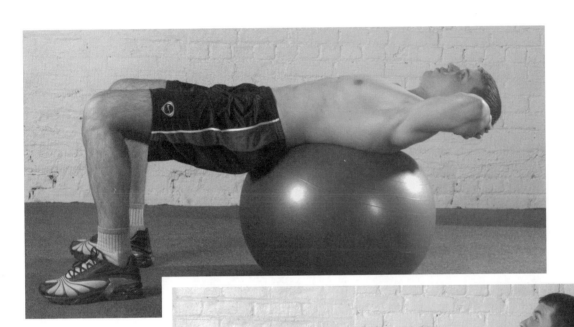

Swiss Ball Reverse Crunch

Great for targeting the lower segment of the *rectus abdominis*, but those of you with lower back trouble may want to take a pass.

TECHNIQUE AND FORM

1 Place a Swiss ball a couple of feet in front of a sturdy object, such as a squat rack, stairway railing, or weight bench.

2 Lie on your back on the ball with your feet flat on the floor and the top of your head pointing toward the sturdy object.

3 Once you feel secure on the ball, reach back and grab the object at the same height as your shoulders.

4 Contract your abs by pulling your belly button toward your spine as you lift your legs off the floor. Keeping your balance on the ball, use your abs and hip flexors to "fold" your legs back onto your torso.

5 Once your legs are as close to your chest as possible, reverse directions and slowly lower your legs back to the starting position.

TRAINER'S TIPS

✪ As you lift your legs toward your chest, simultaneously allow your hips to roll down the ball slightly to intensify the contraction. This mimics the effects of using the abdominal slant board by forcing you to overcome the force of gravity to a greater degree. Ending up directly on top of the ball drastically reduces the effectiveness of the exercise.

✪ Execute the lifting and lowering of the legs in a slow, controlled manner to avoid falling off the ball.

✪ Avoid using your arms to help pull you up on the ball.

✪ When lowering your legs between reps avoid bouncing in the bottom position; make the transition between the lowering and raising phase as smooth as possible.

Swiss Ball Reverse Crunch

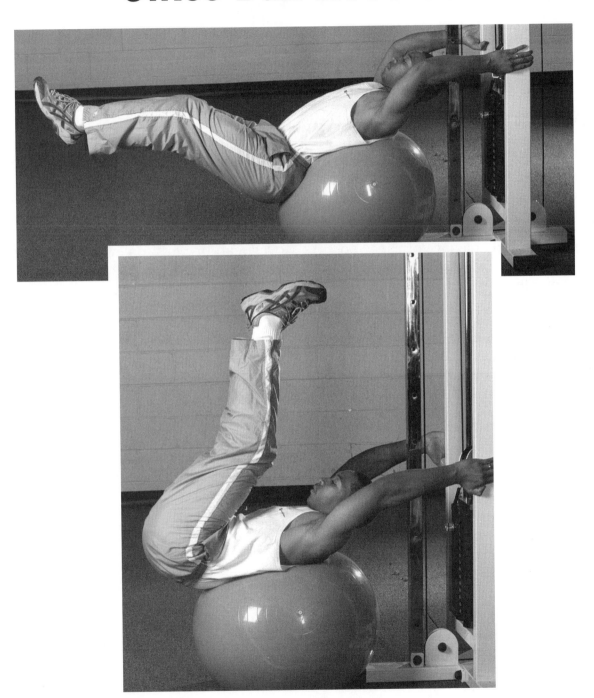

Swiss Ball Oblique Crunch

Once again, the greater range of motion provided by the Swiss ball makes this a more productive exercise.

TECHNIQUE AND FORM

1 Lie sideways on the Swiss ball so that only your right hip and the right side of your rib cage are in contact with it.

2 Place your hands lightly behind your head and scissor your legs so that your right leg is in front of you and your left leg is behind you.

3 Lift your upper body laterally (sideways) off the ball. In the topmost position your abs should be pulled into your spine with your torso flexed laterally toward your left hip.

4 Hold the position momentarily before lowering yourself back to the starting position.

5 Repeat for the desired number of reps before switching to the other side.

TRAINER'S TIPS

❂ The focus here should be on initiating the contraction by bringing your top armpit toward your top hip.

❂ You can make the exercise more challenging by extending your arms overhead or perhaps even holding a medicine ball.

❂ If you find that you are unable to steady yourself on the ball, use a wall to help you. Set the ball up about three feet from the wall and then prop your feet against it to perform the exercise.

Swiss Ball Oblique Crunch

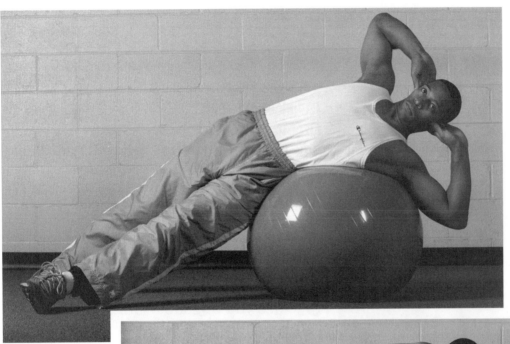

Swiss Ball Circle Crunch

This exercise starts like the standard **Swiss Ball Crunch** (page 68)—but it has an added twist. In this exercise, rather than coming straight up, you arc your torso over the ball.

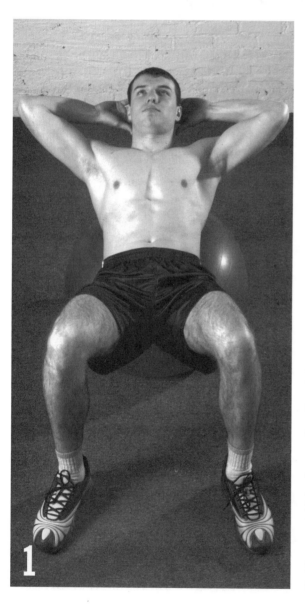

TECHNIQUE AND FORM

1 Lie back on a Swiss ball so that your head is resting on the ball and your back conforms to the ball. Keep your hips slightly lower than your torso and bend your knees at a 90-degree angle.

2 With your hands held behind your head, lift your left shoulder blade off the ball diagonally toward your left.

3 Once you've gone as far left as you can, start lifting your torso up and laterally across to the right side of your body.

4 When you've gone all the way to your right, lower your shoulder blades back down to the ball and repeat by starting on your right side and working toward your left.

5 Repeat for the desired number of reps,

TRAINER'S TIPS

✪ Don't initiate the lift off of the ball by working across your body; when going to your left your left arm and shoulder blade should move first.

✪ To get the feel of the arcing motion, imagine drawing a rainbow over your torso.

Swiss Ball Circle Crunch

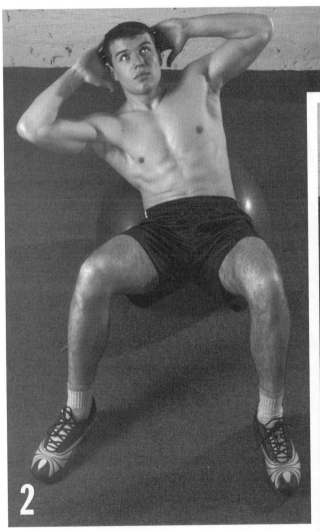

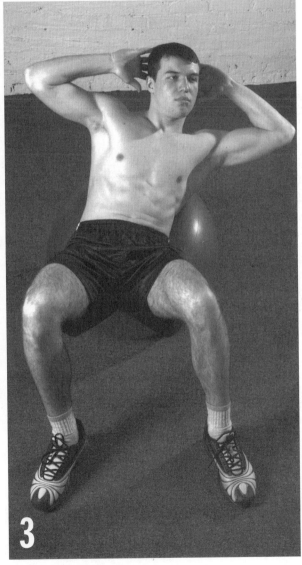

Swiss Ball Crunch With Rotation

Yet another Swiss ball crunch variation—as you can see, the ball offers an almost infinite number of ways to train your abs and core.

TECHNIQUE AND FORM

1 Lie on a Swiss ball with your feet on the floor about shoulder width apart and your knees bent at a 90-degree angle.

2 Making sure your hips are lower than your chest, lie back and allow your back to conform to the ball. With your head cradled in your hands to help support your neck and elbows held out to the sides, crunch your ribcage toward your pelvis by lifting your shoulder blades off the ball.

3 Once your shoulder blades are a couple of inches off the ball, slowly rotate your torso as far to the right as possible and then slowly return to the center and lower yourself back to the starting position.

4 Repeat the same sequence on the other side and continue for the desired number of reps.

TRAINER'S TIPS

✖ Throughout the rotation be sure to keep your elbows back and out of your peripheral vision. Allowing the elbows to pull across the head puts strain on your neck and gives you a false sense of how far you're actually rotating.

✖ Try not to lower out of the crunch position until you've completed the entire rotation.

✖ You'll find that your hips need to shift slightly to allow for complete torso rotation. Therefore, be extra careful to maintain your balance on the ball.

Swiss Ball Crunch with Rotation

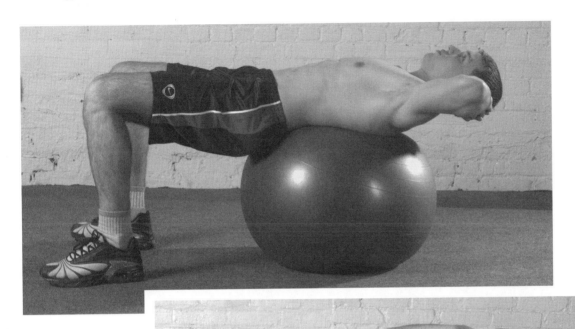

Swiss Ball Corkscrew Crunch

This is another tough one; don't be surprised—or discouraged—if you need to work up to it.

TECHNIQUE AND FORM

1 Set the Swiss ball two to three feet away from a wall. Position yourself on the ball as if you were going to do a Swiss Ball Oblique Crunch (page 72), but brace yourself against the wall with your feet and twist your upper body so that in the starting position your torso is draped over the ball facing the floor.

2 Use your spinal erectors and obliques to initiate your lift off the ball.

3 Once you've reached the midway position of the lift, rotate your torso as much as possible so that at the top of the movement your torso is facing forward and your abs are in a crunched position.

4 Repeat for the desired number of reps.

TRAINER'S TIPS

◈ Perform this exercise in a smooth, controlled manner; avoid abrupt twisting or jerking movements, which can invite injury.

◈ Be sure to keep your abs pulled into your spine throughout the movement to avoid potential strain to your lower back.

Swiss Ball Corkscrew Crunch

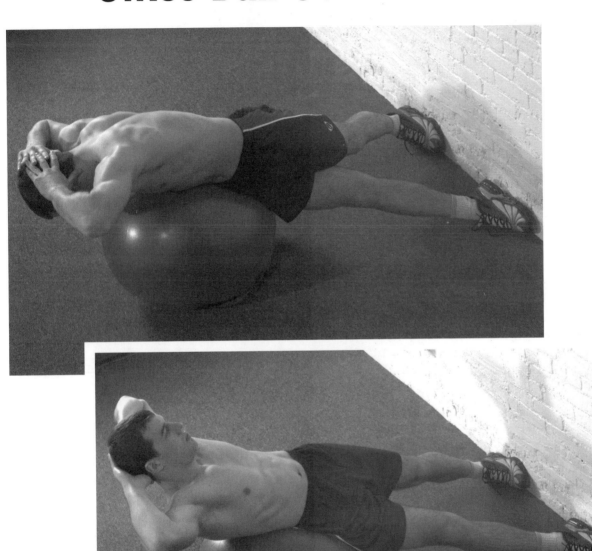

Swiss Ball Bridge

The Swiss Ball Bridge isn't for the faint of heart (or abs). Once you can knock out 30 seconds straight you'll have a seriously strong mid-section.

TECHNIQUE AND FORM

1 Kneel with a Swiss ball in front of you; place your forearms on the ball.

2 Lift your knees off the floor and straighten your legs so that only the balls of your feet are in contact with the floor. Make sure that your back is flat and your pelvis is in a neutral position by pulling your belly button to your spine, hollowing out your waist, and simultaneously tucking in your glutes.

3 Hold this position for 30 to 60 seconds while breathing through pursed lips.

TRAINER'S TIPS

✪ Don't let your hips sag toward the floor at any time during the exercise; doing so will place undo strain on your lower back.

✪ Don't hike your hips up into the air; your body should form a diagonal line from your feet to your head.

✪ Stay propped up on your forearms with your chest away from the ball.

Swiss Ball Bridge

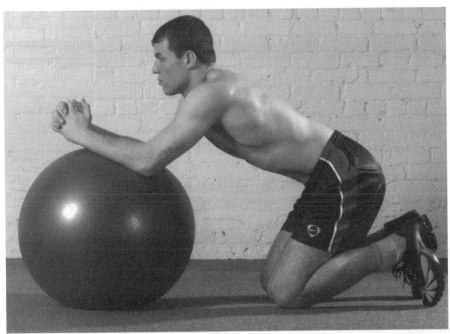

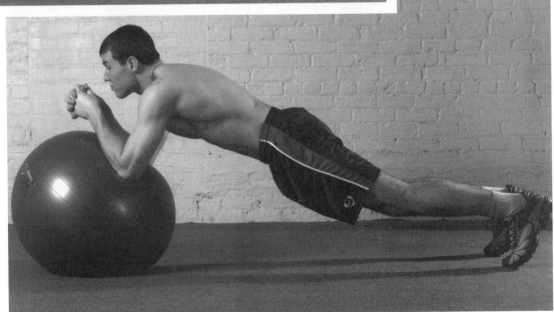

Swiss Ball Jackknife

This one is definitely not for beginners. You'll need to have good upper body strength to stabilize your position on the ball.

TECHNIQUE AND FORM

1 Begin by getting into a push-up position with your feet and lower legs resting on the Swiss ball and your hands on the floor approximately shoulder width apart.

2 Pulling in your abs toward your spine, slowly pull your legs toward your chest by bending your knees and lifting your hips into the air.

3 At the same time, exhale and round your back as much as possible to work your abs.

4 After holding the top position momentarily, slowly straighten your legs and bring the ball back to the starting position.

5 Repeat for the desired number of reps.

TRAINER'S TIPS

In both the starting and finishing position of each rep proper positioning is critical. To avoid strain to the lower back, keep your abs pulled in and your glutes held tight to minimize the arch in your lower back. Allowing your abs to relax and your back to arch excessively can place tremendous strain on your back.

Concentrate on using your abs and hip flexors to pull the ball toward you.

Lift your rear end high into the air and round your back as much as possible to get maximal stimulation out of your abs.

Use a slow, controlled negative to bring the ball back to the starting position; avoid letting it roll away from you quickly.

Swiss Ball Jackknife

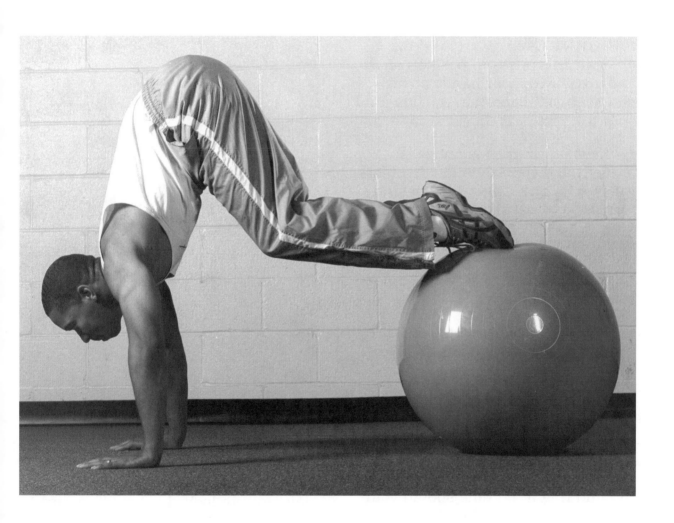

Swiss Ball Lower Body Rotations

This extremely advanced exercise demands some serious upper body strength. Not only that, but you'll also need some pretty strong abs to pull this one off.

TECHNIQUE AND FORM

1 Start in a push-up position on the Swiss ball with your hands about shoulder width apart on the floor and your feet grabbing the sides of the ball.

2 Keeping your arms and legs straight and your abdominals pulled into your spine, allow the ball (and your legs) to roll slowly to one side.

3 When the outside of your foot grazes the floor, use your core muscles to rotate the ball back over to the other side of the floor.

4 Repeat for the desired number of reps.

TRAINER'S TIPS

✪ The position of your pelvis is key to keeping strain off the lower back. Keep your abs pulled in toward your spine throughout the exercise to keep from arching your back too much. And keep in mind that at no time should your hips sag toward the floor.

✪ Lower the ball toward the floor in a controlled manner; don't allow it to just roll over to the side.

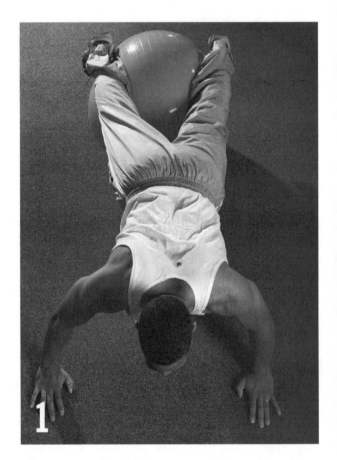

✪ Keep your arms as straight as possible but not locked to avoid undue strain on the elbows.

Swiss Ball Lower Body Rotations

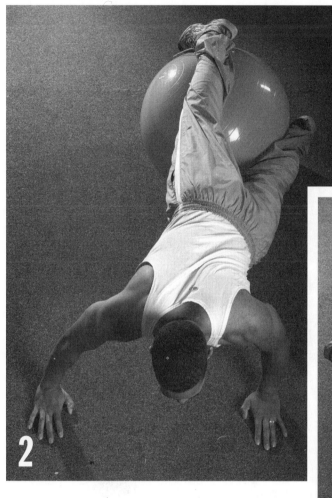

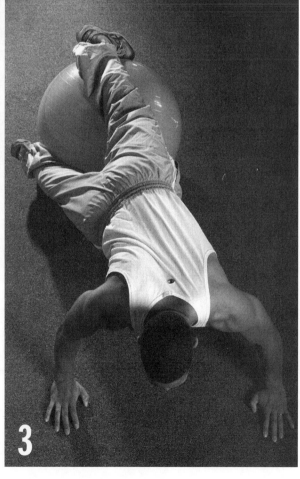

Swiss Ball Figure Eights

This is an *extremely* difficult exercise so be sure to use caution—and don't be surprised if it takes some time to be able to pull if off.

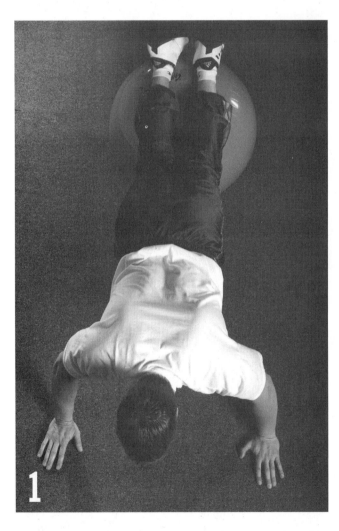

TECHNIQUE AND FORM

1 Begin by getting into a push-up position with your feet and lower legs resting on the Swiss ball and your hands on the floor approximately shoulder width apart.

2 Pull the ball in toward your right armpit.

3 Once you're in the tucked position, stay there and begin to move the ball in a figure 8 pattern: Work the ball over to your left armpit using a small arcing motion and then, using your abs to control the speed of the ball, roll it out on a slight angle to your right. Still holding your abs tight, work the ball over to your left in a slight arc.

4 Repeat for the desired number of reps.

TRAINER'S TIPS

✪ Keep your abs pulled to your spine throughout the exercise.

✪ Try to use your abs, not your legs, to control the ball's path throughout the range of motion.

Swiss Ball Figure Eights

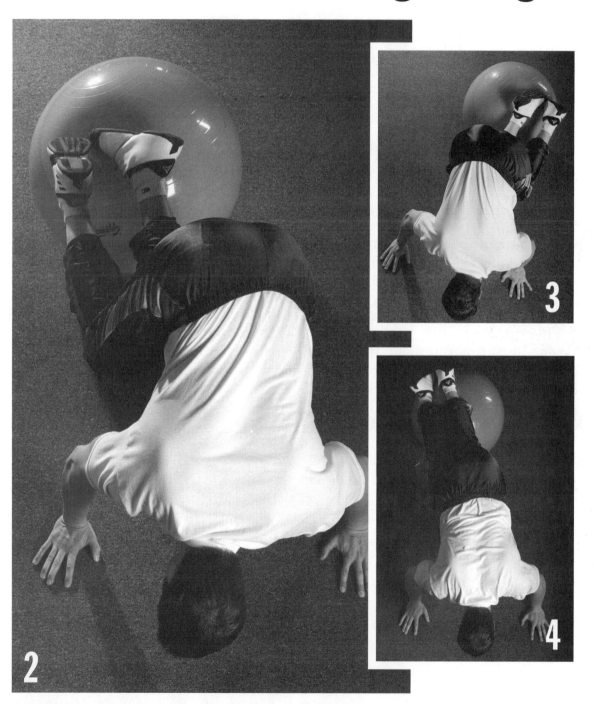

Swiss Ball Pass Off

Don't trust your eyes on this one. It might look easy, but if you perform it correctly, it's an ab-solute gut buster!

TECHNIQUE AND FORM

1 Lie on your back with your arms outstretched behind you and your legs extended straight up and directly over your hips.

2 Holding a Swiss ball between your hands, crunch up, lifting your shoulder blades off the floor, and place the ball between your feet. You're now holding the Swiss ball with your feet.

3 While in the crunch position and leaving your arms outstretched, lower your legs as close to the floor as possible without straining your lower back.

4 Hold that position momentarily before using your abs and hip flexors to bring the ball back up and passing it to your hands.

5 Lower your arms and repeat for the desired number of reps.

TRAINER'S TIPS

As you lower your legs toward the floor, be sure your abs are pulled into your spine. That will minimize the arch in your lower back.

Make sure to lift your shoulder blades off the mat when you're reaching for your feet.

Initiate the arm and leg lift-offs in a controlled manner by contracting the abdominals. Avoid using momentum to propel the ball upward.

Swiss Ball Pass Off

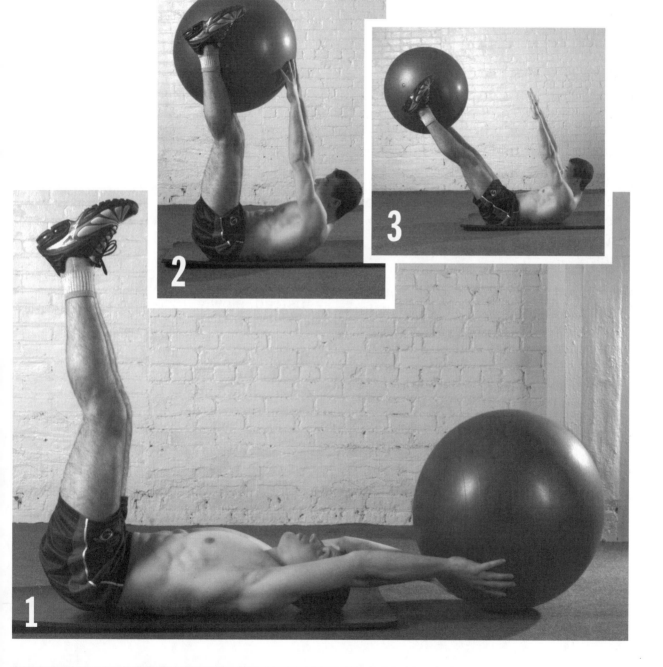

Swiss Ball Cobra

The Swiss Ball Cobra will give your spinal erectors a real workout. Just as with the Swiss Ball Crunch, the increased range of motion increases the difficulty level of the exercise.

TECHNIQUE AND FORM

1 Lie face down on a Swiss ball so that your chest and abdominals are in contact with the ball and your legs are straight, with only the balls of your feet touching the floor.

2 Allow your upper body to curl over the ball and hold your arms out to your sides and bent at 90-degree angles.

3 Uncoil your spine and lift your torso off the ball. As you do so, rotate your arms so that your forearms go from facing behind you at the bottom of the movement to facing in front of you at the top. At the top of the movement your back should be extended with your head, shoulders, and chest lifted off the ball and your arms rotated and even with your head.

4 Lower yourself back to the starting position by returning your arms to their original position as you allow you spine to round over the ball.

5 Repeat for the desired number of reps.

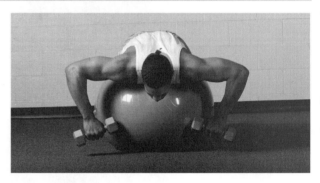

TRAINER'S TIPS

⊗ Be careful not to use momentum to lift your torso up and off of the ball. Instead, slowly uncoil your spine until your back is completely straight.

⊗ Avoid completely relaxing your abs and going into extreme hyperextension when you're in the topmost position. Doing so can place undue strain on your lower back.

⊗ Keep your head pulled back in line with your spine as you extend.

⊗ Avoid jutting your chin forward as you lift up.

⊗ You can make the exercise more challenging by holding a pair of light dumbbells in your hands during this exercise, as shown.

Swiss Ball Cobra

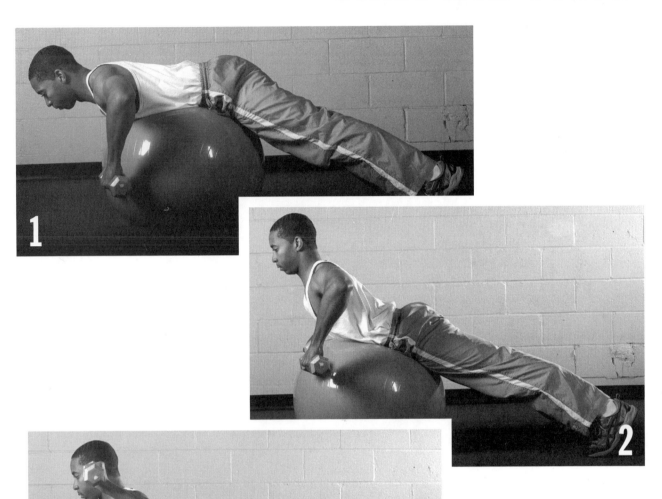

Chapter 6
Medicine Ball Exercises

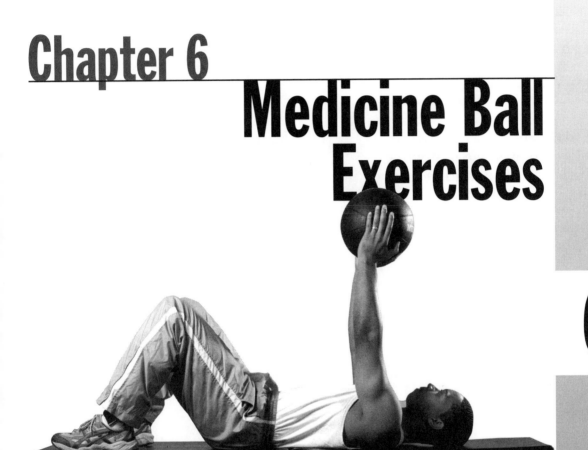

The great thing about working with medicine balls is that they allow you to train your abs for the types of explosive movements you perform during many common sport and leisure activities. Plus, since they're so affordable, they offer an excellent alternative to expensive gym equipment.

6

THE **BODY SCULPTING BIBLE** FOR **ABS**

MEN'S EDITION

Medicine Ball Kneeling Throw

In this drill your abs perform two jobs: (1) they help generate the power you need to throw the ball onto the floor; and (2) they help decelerate your torso so that your momentum doesn't force you forward into a face plant on the mat. You don't need a partner for this exercise—but it's helpful to have someone fetch the ball for you!

TECHNIQUE AND FORM

1 Kneel on an exercise mat while holding an 8- to 12-pound medicine ball between your hands.

2 Extend your arms straight up overhead and pull your abs into your spine.

3 Keeping your arms straight, use your abdominals to quickly and forcefully throw the ball as hard as you can onto the floor about a foot or so in front of you. You should finish with your upper body almost parallel to the floor and your arms extended behind you.

4 Have a partner retrieve the ball for you or get it yourself and repeat the drill for the desired number of reps.

TRAINER'S TIPS

✪ Keep your arms as straight as possible and concentrate on using core power to throw the ball.

✪ Forcibly exhaling as you explode the ball into the floor can increase the intensity of the contraction.

✪ Throw the ball far enough away from you so that it doesn't bounce back up and hit you in the face but not so far as to reduce the effectiveness of the exercise.

Medicine Ball Kneeling Throw

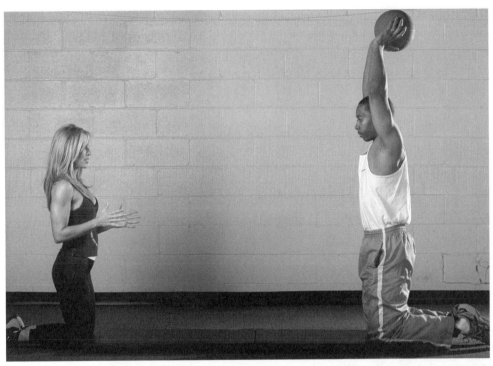

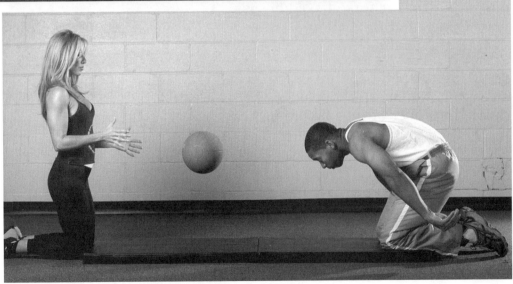

Medicine Ball Woodchopper

Like the Kneeling Throw on the previous page, this exercise requires you to combine an explosive contraction with a rapid deceleration of the abdominals. That means it's important to stand firm and not allow your momentum to move your feet when they're in the bottom position.

TECHNIQUE AND FORM

❶ Stand with your feet shoulder width apart and your knees slightly bent. Hold the medicine ball with your arms extended.

❷ Lift your arms over your left shoulder as you pull your abs into your spine.

❸ Quickly and forcefully "chop" the ball down in a sweeping diagonal motion across your body so that you end up with your torso flexed across your thighs and the ball just outside of your right calf.

❹ Bring the ball back up in the same sweeping motion and repeat for the desired number of reps before switching to the other side.

TRAINER'S TIPS

✪ Keep your arms as straight as possible and focus on sweeping the ball down across your body.

✪ Avoid shortening the movement by bringing the ball only next to your upper thigh; be sure and get it down next to your calf.

Medicine Ball Woodchopper

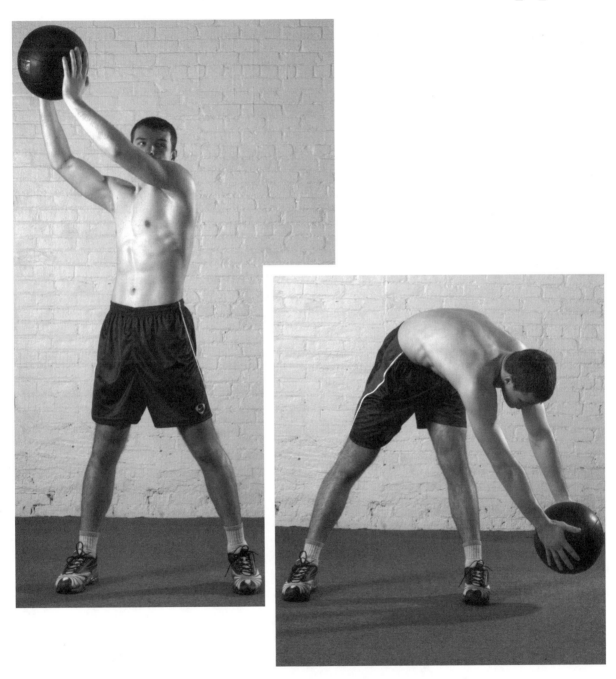

Medicine Ball Overhead Sit-Up

This is an extremely challenging exercise—provided that you don't use momentum to propel your torso off of the floor.

TECHNIQUE AND FORM

1 Lie on your back on an exercise mat. Hold an 8- to 10-pound medicine ball with your arms extended over your head.

2 Keeping your arms straight and the ball directly over your head, sit up until your chest almost touches your thighs.

3 Lower yourself back to the starting position and repeat.

4 Repeat for the desired number of reps.

TRAINER'S TIPS

✪ Avoid "throwing" your upper body forward to generate momentum.

✪ Lower yourself slowly to take advantage of the negative portion of the movement.

✪ Once you've mastered this sit-up with an 8- to 10-pound ball, increase the weight of the medicine ball to 12- to 15 pounds—or heavier.

Medicine Ball Overhead Sit-Up

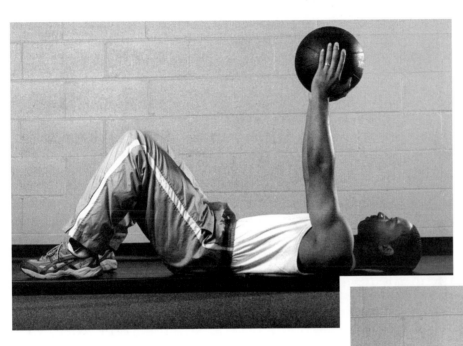

Medicine Ball Bicycle

This one takes a little coordination but the intense abdominal burn you get will be worth the time it takes to learn it.

TECHNIQUE AND FORM

❶ Lie on your back on an exercise mat with your knees slightly bent and only your heels touching the floor.

❷ With your arms extended out to your sides and a 6- to 10-pound medicine ball in one hand, sit up as you simultaneously lift the leg opposite from the hand holding the medicine ball.

❸ As you bring that leg toward your chest, pass the ball under your leg to the opposite arm. As soon as you do, immediately lower yourself back down and repeat to the other side.

❹ Continue for the desired number of reps.

TRAINER'S TIPS

✪ Keep the movement as smooth and fluid as possible.

✪ Avoid resting in the bottom position.

✪ Try to lift both your lower and upper body at the same rate so they meet in the middle.

✪ Use your abs to bring your chest toward your thigh and vice versa. Do not bend and straighten the knees to bring your legs in.

Medicine Ball Bicycle

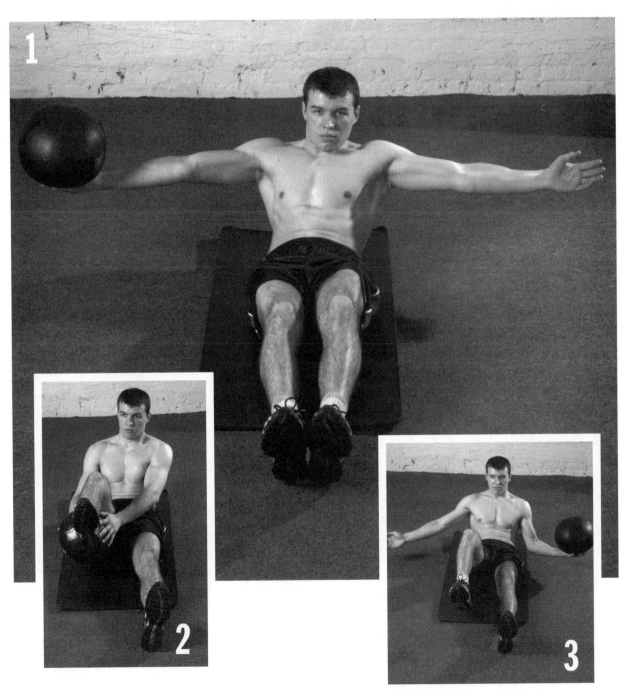

Chapter 7

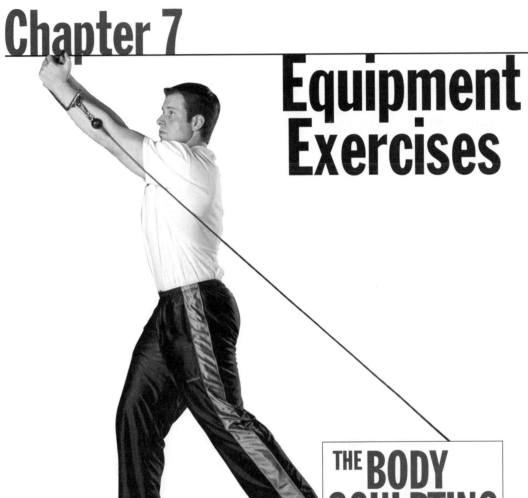

Equipment Exercises

7

THE BODY SCULPTING BIBLE FOR ABS

MEN'S EDITION

Besides Swiss balls and medicine balls, there are lots of other tools you can use to give your abs a great workout. From the inexpensive (barbells) to the more elaborate (cable stations), they can all be used for gut-busting ab exercises.

High-to-Low Cable Woodchopper

An excellent exercise for developing rotational power, the Woodchopper will really put your abs and obliques to work.

TECHNIQUE AND FORM

1 Stand sideways in the middle of a cable station with your feet about shoulder width apart and your knees slightly bent.

2 Reach up and over your left shoulder with both arms and grab hold of the handle attached to the high pulley.

3 Keeping your arms straight and knees slightly bent, bring the weight down in a sweeping, diagonal motion across your body until the cable handle ends up outside your right calf and your torso is flexed across your legs.

4 Slowly reverse direction, returning the weight to the starting position.

5 Repeat for the desired number of reps before switching to the other side.

TRAINER'S TIPS

✦ Keep your arms straight and focus on using your core to pull the weight down and across your body. Avoid pulling the weight with your arms.

✦ Stand firm; try not to move or reposition your feet during the exercise. Stand (and stay) in a ready, athletic stance with your feet apart and knees bent. Generate power with your core, not your legs.

✦ Exhale as you bring the weight down to intensify the contraction.

High-to-Low Cable Woodchopper

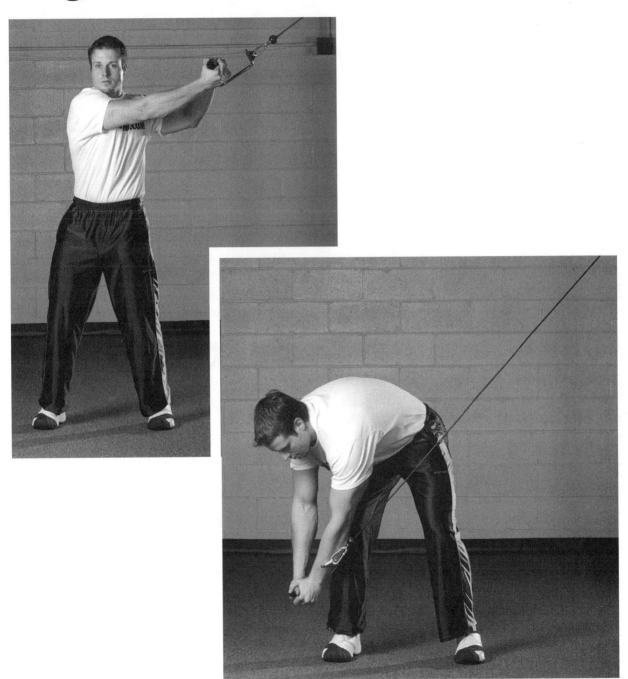

Low-to-High Cable Woodchopper

Another terrific exercise guaranteed to make the toddler in your life very happy. Just make sure you strengthen your abs to the point where you can pick up the little one as often as he or she asks.

TECHNIQUE AND FORM

1 Begin in the same position as for the High-to-Low Woodchopper on the previous page, only this time grab the right *lower* pulley attachment with both hands. Your arms should be straight and your hands positioned just outside your right hip.

2 Keep your shoulders and hips squared and facing forward as you work the weight upward in a sweeping diagonal manner.

3 Once the weight is high over your right shoulder, pause momentarily and then lower the weight back to the starting position.

4 Repeat for the desired number of reps.

TRAINER'S TIPS

❖ Just as you did during the High-to-Low Woodchopper, keep your arms straight throughout the exercise.

❖ Grab the pulley using a hand-over-hand grip. Keep the hand of the side you're going to on the bottom. This helps reduce the tendency to pull the weight with your opposite arm and increases the demand on your core.

❖ Stand firm; try not to shift or move your feet as you perform the exercise.

Low-to-High Cable Woodchopper

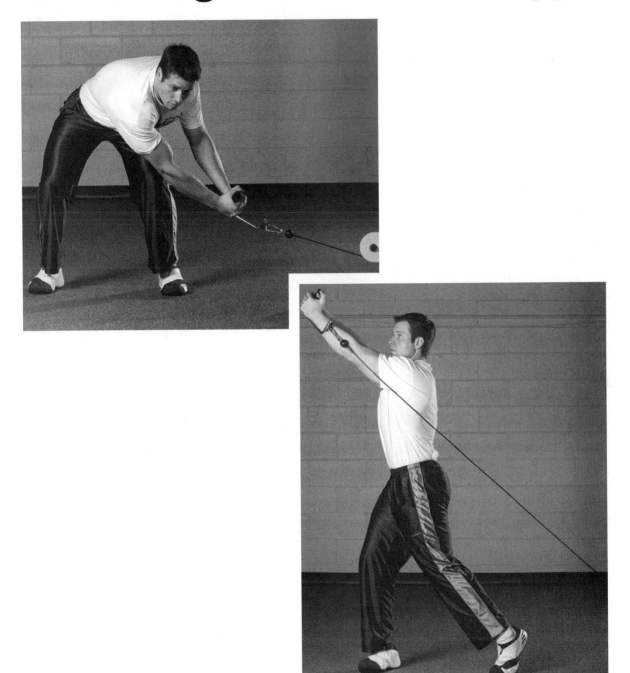

Cable Crunch

This is one of those exercises that people tend to do incorrectly, so make sure to read the Trainer's Tips very carefully.

TECHNIQUE AND FORM

1 Grab the high pulley attachment of the cable station with both hands and then kneel facing the weight stack. You should be a foot or two from the stack.

2 Keeping your elbows slightly bent, tuck your head between your arms and crunch your ribcage toward your pelvis.

3 When your elbows are just about touching the middle of your thighs, slowly uncoil your spine and return to the starting position.

TRAINER'S TIPS

✪ Flexing your spine is the key to this exercise. To do it, imagine someone holding a broomstick horozontally in front of you, about 6 inches away from your belly button. When crunching, imagine bringing your elbows down and over the stick without touching it.

✪ Keep the same degree of bend in your elbows throughout the exercise; don't bend them any more or straighten your arms.

✪ Keep your hips in a fixed position with your rear end off your heels. Don't let them move up and down.

Cable Crunch

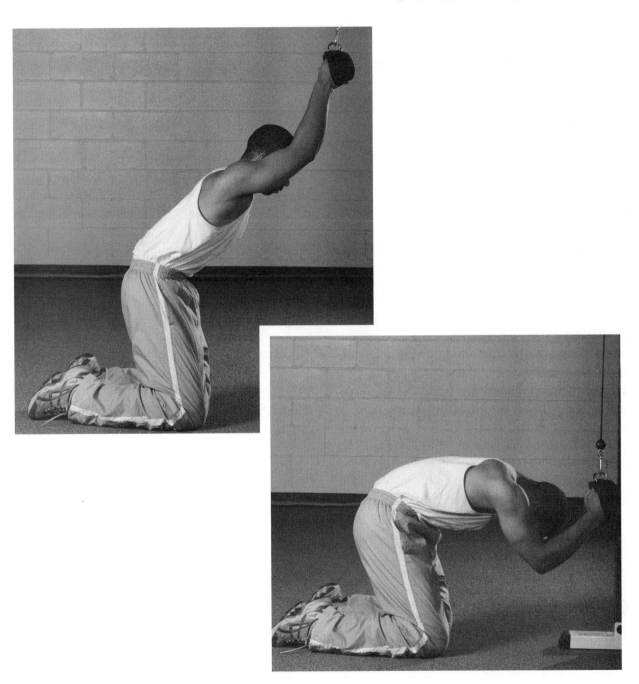

Barbell Rollouts

Are you tough enough for this one? You need to have really good ab and lower back strength before you even *think* about trying it.

TECHNIQUE AND FORM

1 Place one small plate (5- to 10-pounds) at each end of an Olympic barbell; secure with collars.

2 Kneel on an exercise mat, place the bar in front of you horizontally, and grab it with your hands shoulder width apart.

3 With the bar almost touching your knees and your back in a rounded position, let the bar roll out slowly, extending your torso as you do so. Let the bar continue to roll until your arms are just about straight out ahead of you, your entire torso and hips are parallel to the floor, and only your shins and feet are in contact with the floor.

4 Pause momentarily in this bottom position before using your abs to pull you back to the starting position with the bar against your knees and your back rounded.

5 Repeat for the desired number of reps.

TRAINER'S TIPS

As you let the bar roll out and especially in the bottom position, you must maintain a neutral spine by holding in your abs as much as possible and eliminating the arch in your lower back. Otherwise you run the risk of straining your lower back.

Focus on using your abs to initiate the inward pull, don't try to pull the bar back with your arms.

Bring the bar all the way back to your knees and exhale as you round your back to help intensify the contraction.

Barbell Rollouts

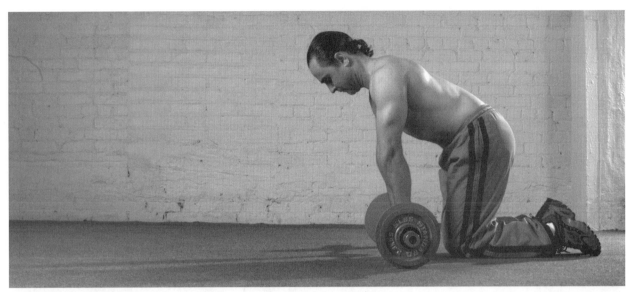

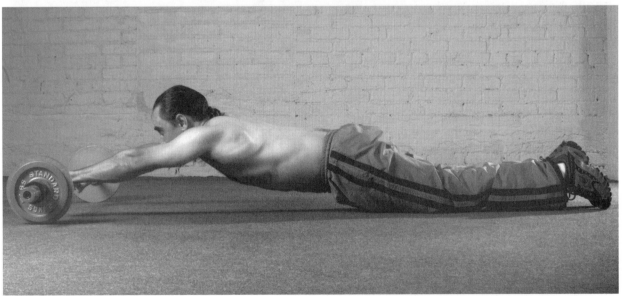

Saxon Side Bends

A word of warning: This exercise is *much* more difficult than the classic side bend, in which you hold a dumbbell at arm's length next to your thigh.

TECHNIQUE AND FORM

1 Grab a pair of lightweight (10- to 12-pound) dumbbells and stand with your feet shoulder width apart and knees slightly bent.

2 Straighten your arms over your head so that the weights line up directly over your shoulders.

3 Pulling your abs to your spine, slowly lean your upper body as far to one side as possible.

4 Once you're leaning over as far as you can, use your abs and obliques to pull yourself back up to the center.

5 Repeat on the other side and then continue for the desired number of reps.

TRAINER'S TIPS

The most common error you can make is to rotate your torso as you lean. Keep the movement lateral by making sure your shoulders and hips face forward at all times—no twisting.

Avoid locking your knees (keep them soft), arching your back (maintain neutral spine), or bending and straightening your arms (keep them straight).

You can use a medicine ball in place of weights for this exercise. Hold one ball with both hands over your head.

Saxon Side Bends

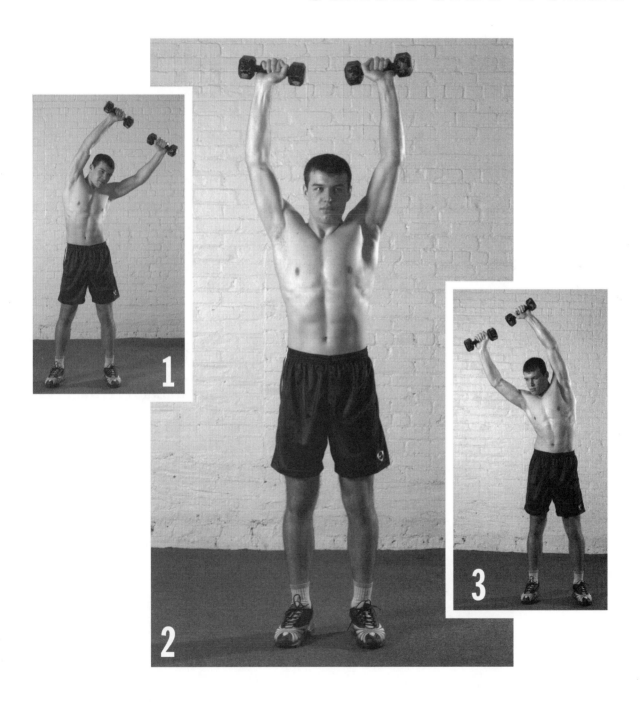

Hanging Leg Raises

This is probably the number one ab exercise that is most often performed incorrectly. That's because most people lack the strength to do the exercise the right way. Keep it up and you'll get there.

TECHNIQUE AND FORM

1 Place your upper arms in a pair of Ab-Originals™ and hang from an overhead bar.

2 Without swinging, use your abs and hip flexors to pull your legs up and in toward your chest.

3 As you do so, round your back and pull your thighs in as close to your chest as possible.

4 Exhale at the top of the motion and then slowly lower your legs to the starting position.

5 Repeat for the desired number of reps.

TRAINER'S TIPS

✪ Avoid swinging your body back and forth to build the momentum to lift your legs.

✪ Spinal flexion is key here. That means you have to lift your legs high enough so that your hips "roll" under your body slightly and your back rounds.

✪ Keeping your back straight and lifting only your knees places far too much emphasis on the hip flexors and works your abdominals only minimally.

✪ Lower your legs to the bottom position only to the point at which you can maintain a neutral pelvis. This will help keep tension on your abs and off of your lower back.

Hanging Leg Raises

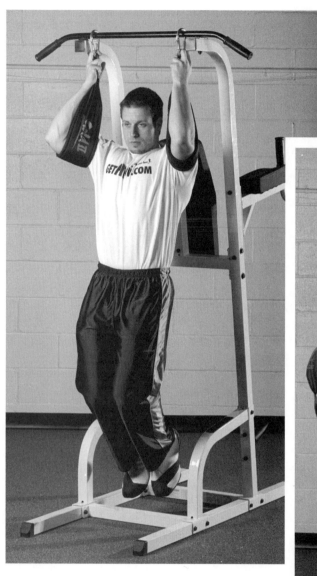

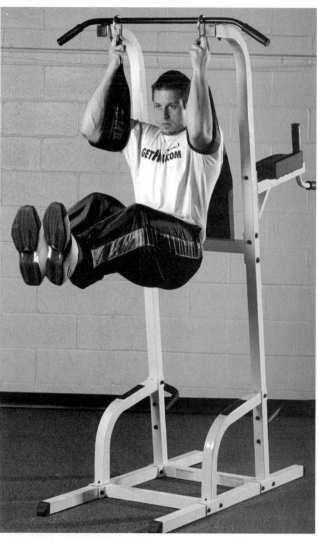

Hanging Oblique Raise

If you thought the Hanging Leg Raises were tough get ready, because this one will knock your socks off.

TECHNIQUE AND FORM

1 Get into the Ab-Originals™ as if you were going to perform Hanging Leg Raises. This time, however, keep your back straight as you lift your knees until your upper thighs are parallel to the floor.

2 Holding that position, slowly lift your right hip toward your right armpit.

3 Once you're as high as you can go, pause momentarily before lowering yourself back to the original position and proceed to the other side.

4 Repeat for the desired number of reps.

TRAINER'S TIPS

✦ Concentrate on using your obliques to pull your hip up toward your armpits.

✦ Keep your knees bent as you lower yourself; don't let your legs straighten between reps. Only after completing a full set of reps should you lower your legs.

✦ When you're in the contracted position, your shins should be diagonal to the floor.

Hanging Oblique Raise

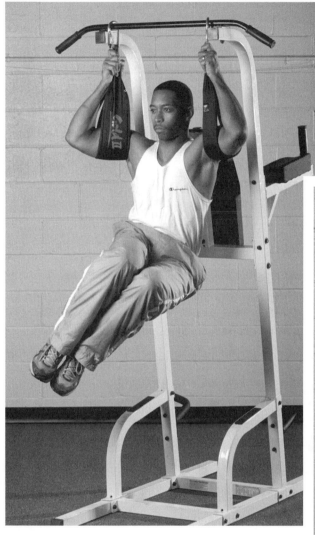

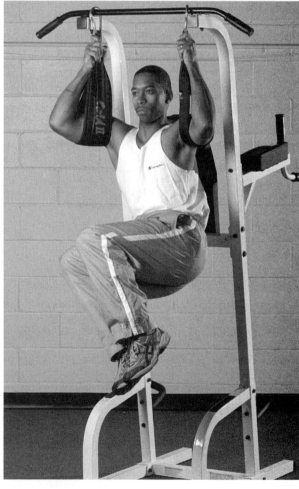

Slant Board Reverse Crunch

When you do this exercise, think of folding your body in half at the waist; avoid just bending and straightening your legs.

TECHNIQUE AND FORM

1 Lie on an abdominal slant board or decline weight bench with your arms extended above your head. Hold the back of the bench for support.

2 Lift your legs so that your knees are above your hips and your legs form a 90-degree angle.

3 Slowly lift your legs toward your chest, making sure to round your lower back and lift your tailbone off of the bench as you do so. In the contracted position, your thighs should be almost touching your chest with your lower back rounded.

4 Hold that position momentarily before lowering yourself back to the starting position.

5 Repeat for the desired number of reps.

TRAINER'S TIPS

The key in this exercise—as in many of the others—is spinal flexion. Pulling in your legs just by bending your knees will do little for your abs. Think of your pelvis as a bowl of water that you're dumping out onto your chest to get a feel for how to flex your spine.

The difficulty of this exercise depends on the steepness of the incline. The steeper the incline, the more you have to overcome the effects of gravity.

Don't lift your back too high off the bench. Lifting your lower back slightly should give you all the spinal flexion you need.

Slant Board Reverse Crunch

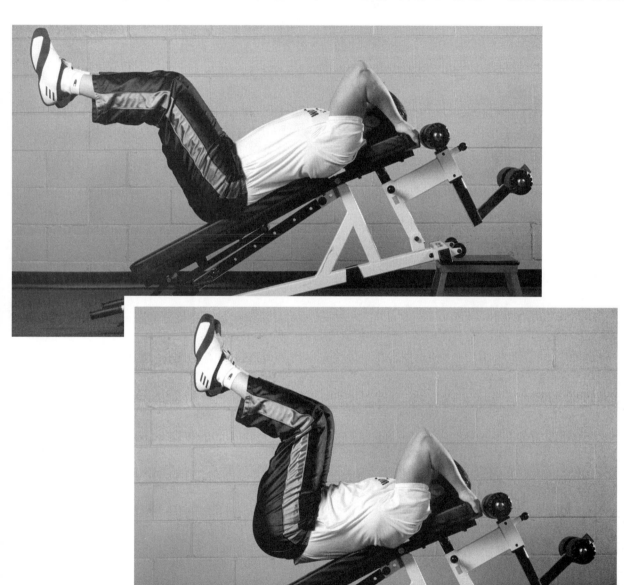

The Drawbridge

This is a super advanced exercise—so please use caution.

TECHNIQUE AND FORM

1 There are two ways to perform this exercise and both start from the same position: Lie back on an exercise bench with your legs slightly bent. Hold the end of the bench behind your head.

2 Lift your legs into the air over your hips and then slowly roll your weight back onto your shoulder blades.

3 Once there, lift your legs toward the ceiling as high as possible before slowly lowering your body toward the surface of the bench. Be sure to keep your body straight and your abs pulled into your spine as you lower yourself in a slow, controlled manner.

4 Once you're as close to the bench as you can get you can do one of two things: Gently lower yourself all the way back to the starting position described in Step 1 and then repeat the exercise; or if you're strong enough, lower yourself back to the position described in Step 2, and then pull yourself back up.

5 Repeat for the desired number of reps.

TRAINER'S TIPS

◆ It's vital to keep your abs pulled to your spine to support your back throughout the exercise.

The Drawbridge

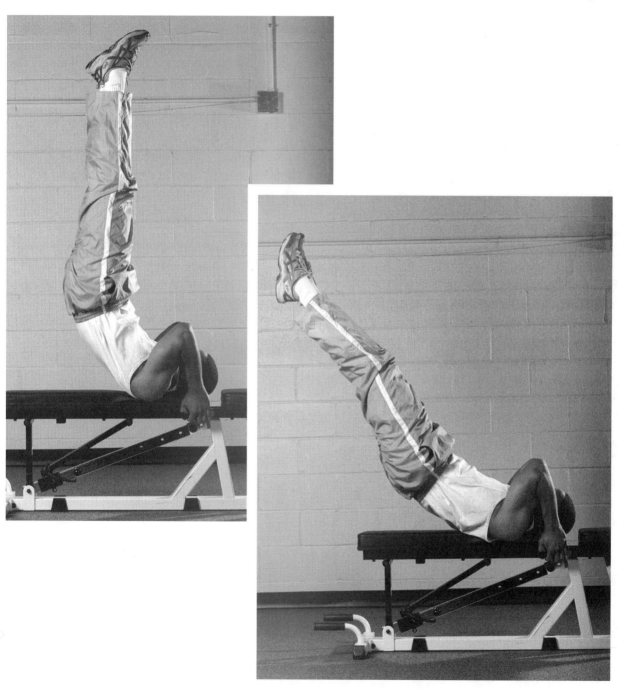

Full-Contact Twists

This is a great exercise for improving your striking power for martial arts or sports such as tennis.

TECHNIQUE AND FORM

1 Prop the end of a barbell in the corner of a squat rack or the corner of a room.

2 Grab the bar with your arms straight and fingers interlocked, holding the bar at about a 45 degree angle to the floor.

3 With your feet about shoulder width apart and knees bent, quickly work the bar over to one side in an arcing motion until it's in line with your left hip. Be sure to pivot your feet as you do so and turn your toes in the same direction you're facing to avoid sheering force on your knees.

4 Quickly work the bar up and over to the other side using your core musculature to generate the necessary power.

TRAINER'S TIPS

Pivoting the feet is crucial to avoiding knee injury.

Keep your arms straight and focus on using core power to move the barbell.

Do not allow the weight to pull your torso over to the side in the bottom position; remain as upright as possible.

Full-Contact Twists

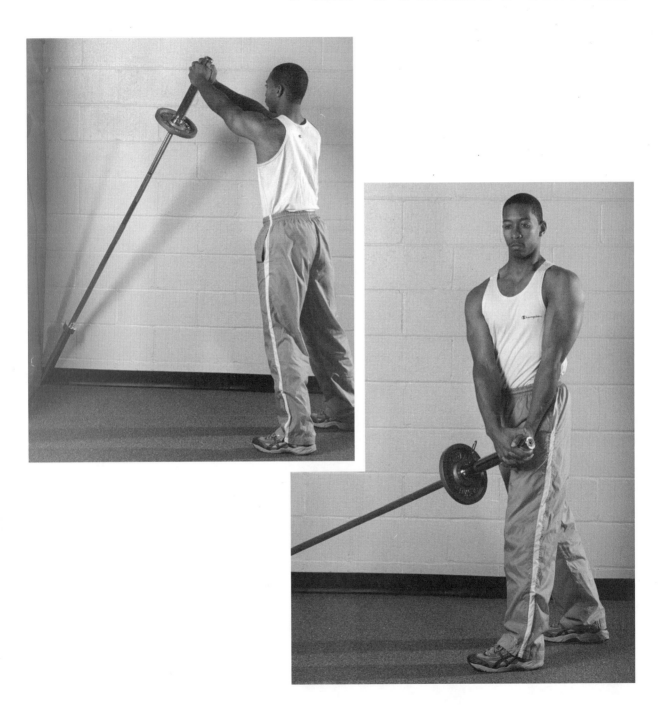

Chapter 8
Lower Back Exercises

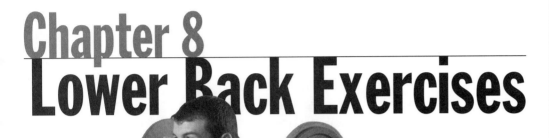

The following six exercises not
only train your lower back, but
they also make your entire
core work hard. For example,
the Overhead Squat involves
no quick movements, but it
places incredible demands
on your lower back mus-
cles to help stabilize your
position—not to mention the
amount of work your abs are
forced to do to stabilize the
bar. It is this ability to force
your abs and lower back to
work together as a unit that
makes these exercises so
tremendously benefi-
cial from a practical
standpoint. Since you
will rarely, if ever, isolate your
abs or lower back during everyday activities, you need to include some
integrated exercises to prepare yourself
for the unique demands imposed by
just living your life.

8

THE **BODY
SCULPTING
BIBLE**
FOR **ABS**

MEN'S EDITION

Supermans

If you work your abs, you've got to work your lower back, too. Here's a simple but effective exercise to target those often-ignored spinal erectors—the muscles that support your spinal column.

TECHNIQUE AND FORM

❶ Lie flat on your stomach on the exercise mat. Extend your arms straight out in front of you and your legs straight out behind you.

❷ Keeping your arms and legs perfectly straight, simultaneously lift your arms, chest, and legs a few inches off the mat.

❸ Once there, hold the position for a second or two before lowering again.

❹ Repeat the exercise for the desired number of reps.

TRAINER'S TIPS

✦ Make sure that you lift yourself off of the mat in a slow, controlled manner; avoid jerking yourself up into position.

✦ Try to look at the floor throughout the movement to avoid unnecessary hyperextension of the neck.

✦ For an effective variation of this exercise, begin in the same starting postion described in Step 1. Next, simultaneously lift your right arm and left leg off the floor. Switch arms/legs and repeat.

✦ You can even perform the exercise on all fours, lifting and extending your left arm and right leg and vice versa.

Supermans

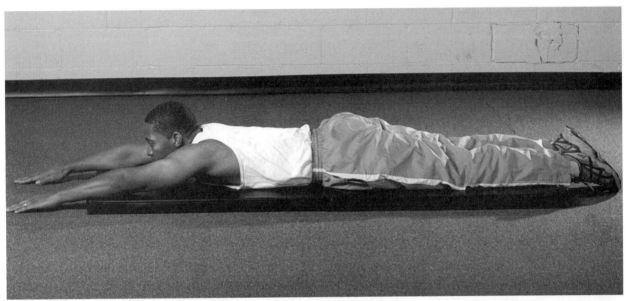

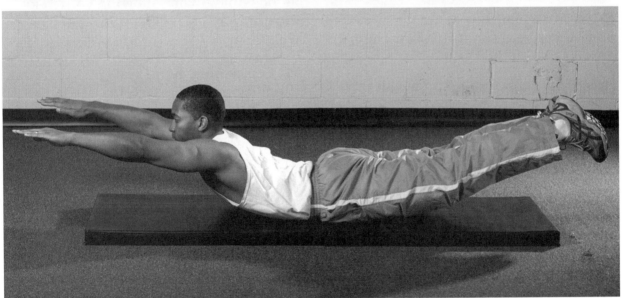

Dead Lifts

Quite simply one of the best exercises you can do. Trouble is, few people ever do them! It's time for you to break the mold.

TECHNIQUE AND FORM

1 Stand holding a barbell with a pronated (palms facing down) grip. Your feet should be shoulder width apart and your knees slightly bent.

2 Keeping your arms completely straight, lower the bar by bending at your knees and hips so that your hips stick out behind you slightly and your torso remains as upright as possible.

3 Maintaining that same torso position, lower yourself until your thighs are parallel to the floor.

4 Pause momentarily and then change directions, slowly rising again to a standing position.

5 Repeat for the desired number of reps.

TRAINER'S TIPS

● Keep the bar as close to you as possible throughout the entire range of motion by scraping your thighs, knees, and your shins with the bar.

● Don't allow the bar to drift too far in front of you; it increases the strain on your lower back.

● Maintain an upright torso as much as possible; avoid allowing your back to round as you lower and raise the weight.

● Focus on driving your feet through the floor to lift the weight.

● Maintain a slight arch in your lower back and keep your abs pulled to your spine throughout the lift.

Dead Lifts

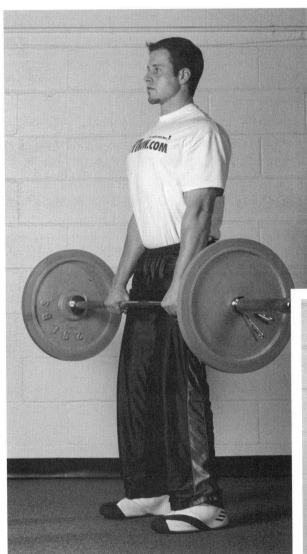

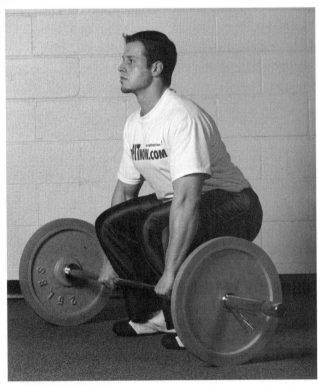

Overhead Squats

You may need to work on improving your flexibility before you can execute this movement properly.

TECHNIQUE AND FORM

1 Grab a barbell with an overhand grip. Your hands should be about twice your shoulder width apart.

2 With your feet about shoulder width apart and knees slightly bent, press the bar up overhead until your arms are completely straight.

3 Keeping the bar overhead, slowly lower yourself into a squat until your thighs are parallel to the floor. Once there, pause momentarily before bringing the weight back up to the starting position.

4 Continue for the desired number of reps.

TRAINER'S TIPS

❂ Make sure that your arms stay as straight as possible throughout the lift and that your arms stay just beyond your peripheral vision. Allowing your arms to drift forward can increase strain on the upper and lower back.

❂ Keep your abs pulled to your spine throughout the lift and especially in the bottom position.

Overhead Squats

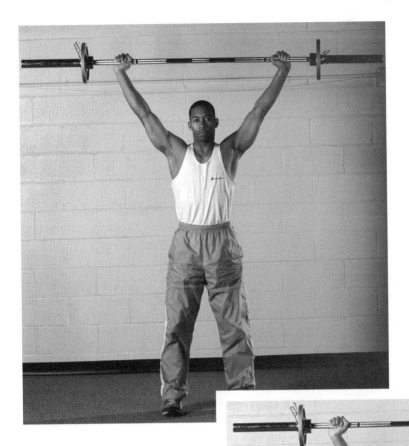

Good Mornings

This is a very advanced exercise—but when performed correctly a terrific one—so please use caution. You need to fully concentrate on your form as you do the Good Mornings to get the full benefit and avoid injury.

TECHNIQUE AND FORM

❶ Place a barbell across your upper back so that it rests on your upper trapezius, just above your shoulder blades.

❷ With your feet about shoulder width apart and knees slightly bent, lean forward, breaking at the hips, until your torso is just about parallel to the ground. Pause momentarily before bringing the bar back up to the starting position.

❸ Repeat for the desired number of reps.

TRAINER'S TIPS

◆ Concentrate during every single rep of this exercise; losing your alignment could lead to injury.

◆ Keep your shoulder blades together and your chest out throughout the exercise.

◆ Try not to alter the amount of bend in your knees as you raise and lower the weight. Start with a slight bend in your knees and concentrate on using the hips as the fulcrum of the movement.

◆ It is crucial that you maintain an arch in your lower back as you lower and raise the weight. Allowing your back to round when your spine is flexed forward greatly increases your risk of injury.

◆ Concentrate on driving your heels into the floor to lift the weight back up. Do not try and simply extend your spine.

Good Mornings

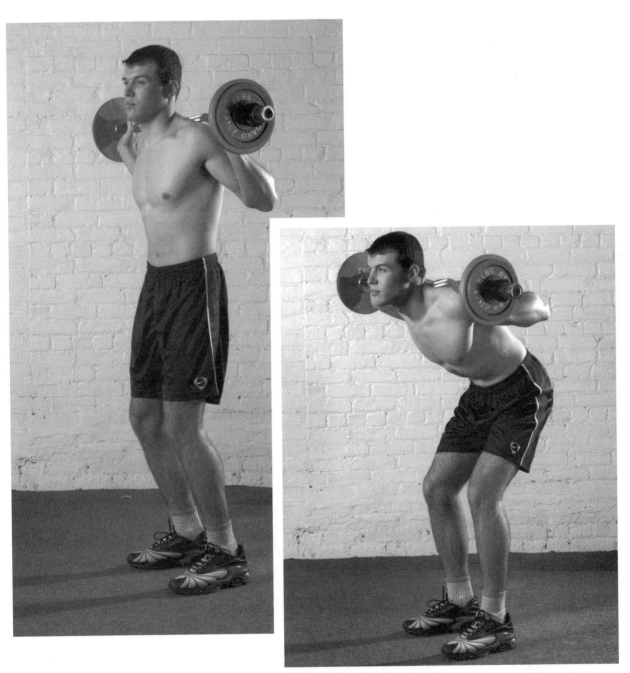

Suitcase Dead Lifts

The Suitcase Dead Lift is aptly titled; but it can be a bit awkward to perform, so you may need to start with a lighter weight than you can actually lift to get a feel for the balance required. The key to this exercise is to lift the weight as if both sides of your body were equally loaded.

TECHNIQUE AND FORM

❶ Grab a barbell in the middle of its bar with one hand—as if you were picking up a suitcase. Stand with your feet shoulder width apart and knees slightly bent.

❷ Slowly squat with the bar, keeping your torso as erect as possible.

❸ Once you've descended to the point where your thighs are parallel to the floor, pause momentarily before pressing back up to the starting position.

❹ Repeat for the desired number of reps before moving the barbell to the opposite hand.

TRAINER'S TIPS

✪ Keep your shoulders and hips squared forward; do not allow the arm holding the dumbbell to pull into a lopsided posture.

✪ Keep you abs pulled to your spine and maintain a slight arch in your lower back throughout the exercise.

Suitcase Dead Lifts

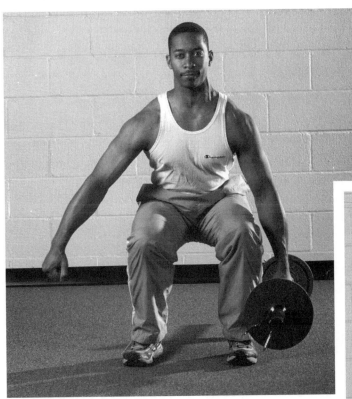

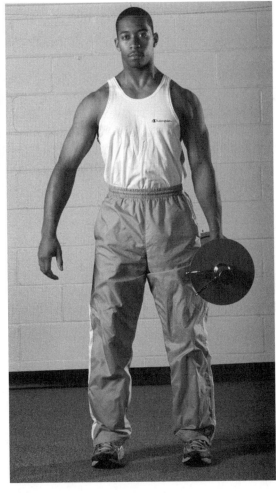

Unilateral Romanian Dead Lift

This one's almost as difficult to perform as it is to say. Once you get it down however, you can just feel that it's doing your body some good.

TECHNIQUE AND FORM

1 Stand with your feet about shoulder width apart and knees slightly bent.

2 Keeping your torso straight and tall, lift one foot an inch or two off of the floor.

3 Once you feel balanced, maintain a slight bend in the other knee as you slowly lean forward by sticking your hips back and bringing your torso over toward the floor. As you descend, be sure to maintain the arch in your lower back.

4 Once your torso is just about parallel to the floor, pause momentarily before lifting back up into the starting position.

5 Repeat for the desired number of reps.

TRAINER'S TIPS

❂ Keep the non-working leg about an inch or two from the floor throughout the exercise. Don't let it lean against the other leg for support.

❂ Maintain a slight arch in your back throughout the exercise.

❂ Do not allow your back to round at any point during the lift.

❂ Allow your arms to hang straight down beneath your shoulders. Once you've mastered the lift with just your body weight, perform the exercise with some light dumbbells in your hands.

Unilateral Romanian Dead Lift

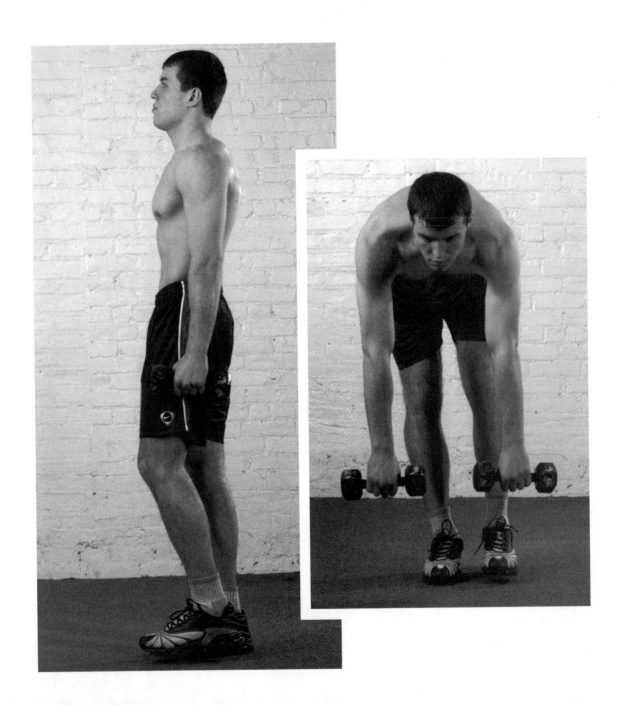

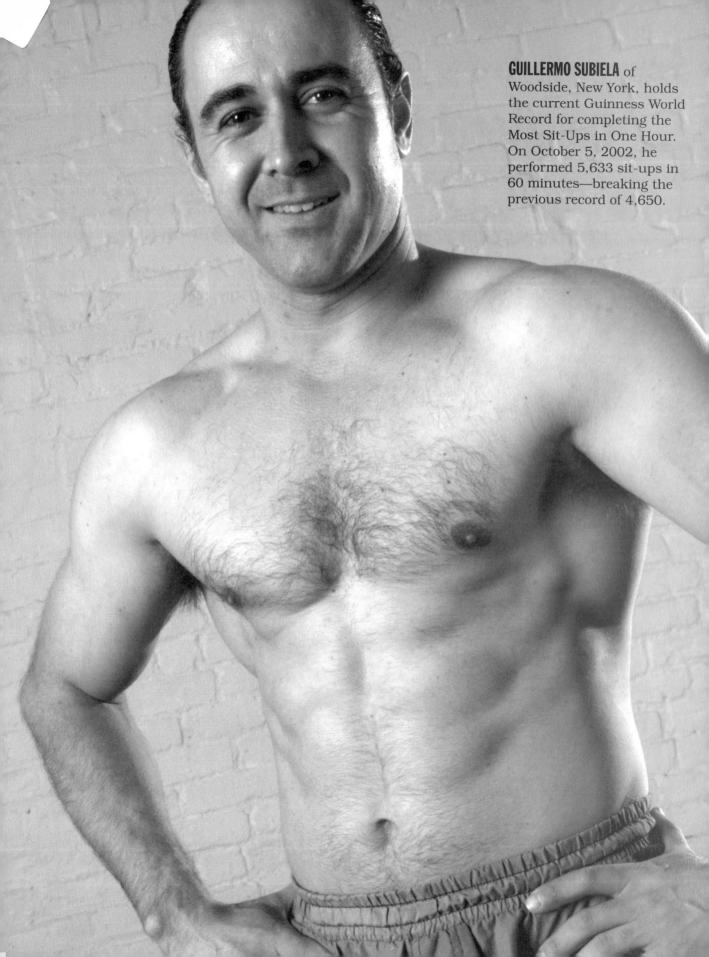

GUILLERMO SUBIELA of Woodside, New York, holds the current Guinness World Record for completing the Most Sit-Ups in One Hour. On October 5, 2002, he performed 5,633 sit-ups in 60 minutes—breaking the previous record of 4,650.

Part 3

THE BODY SCULPTING BIBLE FOR ABS
14-DAY WORKOUTS

THE BODY SCULPTING BIBLE FOR ABS

MEN'S EDITION

Chapter 9
The Workouts

Whether you're just starting out or are already on your way to steel-belted abs, there's a workout here for you. We've even included an Ab Workout To Go that you can do on vacation or a business trip.

9

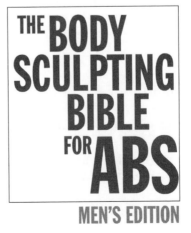

THE **BODY**
SCULPTING
BIBLE
FOR **ABS**
MEN'S EDITION

GETTING STARTED

You want a rippling six-pack? You've come to the right place. It won't happen overnight and it's going to take a lot of work, dedication, consistency, and intensity on your part. But with our 14-Day Ab Sculpting Workouts, you'll be off to a good start.

All of our workouts were designed to be as user friendly as possible. We've set them in chart format, so that you can Xerox the pages and take them to the gym with you.

We've also included the page numbers of the exercises in the chart to make it easy to refer back to the photographs and descriptions.

First things first. If you haven't been doing much—or any—ab work lately, you'll want to start your program with the 14-Day Break-In Workouts. They were designed to get your gut up and running, so to speak; to ready you for the more intense work to come.

Already in pretty good shape? Go ahead and start with the 14-Day Ab Sculpting Workouts. These more advanced programs are your ticket to ripped, chiseled, washboard abs.

SCHEDULING YOUR AB WORKOUTS

When should you do your ab training? There are several answers to that question. If abs are your priority, do these workouts prior to your strength training work or on a separate day. Otherwise, you can do them after your strength work—though with the intensity level increasing, that's going to be pretty tough in the later weeks.

THE BREAK-IN WORKOUTS

Here's what you can expect from the 14-Day Break-In Workouts:

You'll do abs work on three (non-consecutive) days a week for at least two weeks.

If you haven't already, you'll need to start incorporating two to three total-body strength workouts into your schedule as well as two to three days of interval cardio work.

Start each of your workouts with an overall total-body warm-up and then progress to the specific warm-ups on pages 26 to 43.

If, after two weeks, you don't feel ready to move on, don't. Just repeat the 14-Day Break-In Routine for another several weeks.

THE 14-DAY ABS SCULPTING WORKOUTS

Here's the low-down on these workouts:

There are two workouts, Level I and Level II. Each workout is comprised of a six-week program that has been broken down into 14-day segments. That means in each level you'll do six weeks of abs work, changing the specific workouts every two weeks.

The workouts have been designed to be progressive, becoming more difficult as the week progress. That means you need to do them in order—Level I first and then Level II—with no skipping around.

By the end of the first six weeks, you should be feeling and seeing significant results *as long as you've also been following a sound diet and incorporating interval cardio work into your life.*

Level II is an advanced workout. (That does not mean the Level I exercises are "easy," as you will discover.) So if you're not able to perform the exercises with proper form—and proper form is of paramount importance— repeat the previous 14-day workout.

You'll notice that as the weeks progress you're actually doing fewer reps. What's up? As the number of reps decrease you'll need to add resistance. That could mean, for example, using a heavier medicine ball for the Woodchoppers, holding a plate on your chest

THE ZONE-TONE METHOD

The mind-to-muscle connection, coupled with proper exercise technique and form, are crucial if you want to stimulate the necessary muscle fibers needed to create dynamite abs. That may sound like common sense, but most people neglect the mental aspect of training. How about you? When you're getting ready to do an exercise, do you ever stop to think about exactly what muscles you're about to train? Well, you should, because it really will increase the effectiveness of any exercise you do. I've designed a technique, called the Zone-Tone Method, that will help you do just that.

The Zone-Tone method helps you to mentally focus on and preisolate specific muscles just before and during an exercise. The technique is easy to grasp and will deliver enormous benefits to your fitness program. Combining proper form and technique with the Zone-Tone method will help you reach your goals more quickly.

There are only two simple steps to the Zone-Tone method:

❶ Zone in on the individual muscles you intend to train before you begin the exercise. Before each set, before each rep, concentrate on the individual muscles you'll be working. Now tense and flex that muscle as hard as comfortably possible before performing the exercise. What you're doing is preparing the muscle by isolating it even before the exercise begins. This is making the mind-to-muscle connection.

❷ Maintain your mind-to-muscle connection during the exercise. Feel the muscle elongate (stretch) and contract and flex the muscle as hard as you can as you did in Step 1 (except now you flex during the exercise). This is crucial; there's no point in activating the muscles before the exercise begins if you don't do it during the exercise, too.

Most people waste their time by exercising without thinking about what they're doing. That's fine if you're content with average results, but who wants to be average? On the other hand, if you want to compound your efforts exponentially, then you must effectively develop the mind-to-muscle connection. I guarantee that if you use this Zone-Tone technique with the 14-Day Ab Sculpting Workout, you'll achieve better results in less time.

as you do the Slow Sit-Ups, or wearing ankle weights and holding light dumbbells while you do the Supermans. In every instance, the weight needs to be heavy enough that you can just complete the given number of reps, but not so heavy that it screws up your form.

One last thing. Before you get started, you should review the principles of my Zone-Tone training technique, which I laid out in *The Body Sculpting Bible for Men*. There's a short refresher above.

Break-In Workout: Week 1

SPECIAL INSTRUCTIONS FOR WEEKS 1 & 2

- Perform three ab workouts each week.
- Begin to incorporate two to three total-body strength workouts and two to three days of interval cardio in your program.
- Start with a general warm-up and then proceed to the Ab Warm-Ups (pages 26 to 43) before beginning these workouts.

DAY 1			
No.	**Exercise**	**Page No.**	**Reps/Time**
1	Slow Sit-Up	56	8 to 10
2	Oblique V-Up	54	6 to 8 on each side
3	Slant Board Reverse Crunch	118	10 to 12
4	Supermans	126	10 to 12

Perform as a circuit (one exercise after the other).

DAY 2			
No.	**Exercise**	**Page No.**	**Reps/Time**
1	Twisting Pulse-Up	64	6 to 8 on each side
2	Towel Crunch	48	12 to 15
3	Medicine Ball Woodchopper	96	6 to 8 on each side
4	Vacuum	46	6 to 10

Perform as a circuit (one exercise after the other).

DAY 3			
No.	**Exercise**	**Page No.**	**Reps/Time**
1	Slow Sit-Up	56	8 to 10
2	Oblique V-Up	54	6 to 8 on each side
3	Slant Board Reverse Crunch	118	10 to 12
4	Supermans	126	10 to 12

Perform as a circuit (one exercise after the other).

Break-In Workout: Week 2

SPECIAL INSTRUCTIONS FOR WEEKS 1 & 2

- Perform three ab workouts each week.
- Begin to incorporate two to three total-body strength workouts and two to three days of interval cardio in your program.
- Start with a general warm-up and then proceed to the Ab Warm-Ups (pages 26 to 43) before beginning these workouts.

No.	DAY 1 Exercise	Page No.	Reps/Time
1	Twisting Pulse-Up	64	6 to 8 on each side
2	Towel Crunch	48	12 to 15
3	Medicine Ball Woodchopper	96	6 to 8 on each side
4	Vacuum	46	6 to 10

Perform as a circuit (one exercise after the other).

No.	DAY 2 Exercise	Page No.	Reps/Time
1	Slow Sit-Up	56	8 to 10
2	Oblique V-Up	54	6 to 8 on each side
3	Slant Board Reverse Crunch	118	10 to 12
4	Supermans	126	10 to 12

Perform as a circuit (one exercise after the other).

No.	DAY 3 Exercise	Page No.	Reps/Time
1	Twisting Pulse-Up	64	6 to 8 on each side
2	Towel Crunch	48	12 to 15
3	Medicine Ball Woodchopper	96	6 to 8 on each side
4	Vacuum	46	6 to 10

Perform as a circuit (one exercise after the other).

14-Day Ab Sculpting Workout #1: Weeks 1 & 2

SPECIAL INSTRUCTIONS FOR WEEKS 1 & 2

- Perform three ab workouts each week. Incorporate two to three total-body strength workouts and two to three days of interval cardio in your program.
- Start with a general warm-up and then proceed to the Ab Warm-Ups (pages 26 to 43) before beginning these workouts.

DAY 1			FOCUS: CORE STABILITY AND STRENGTH	
No.	**Exercise**	**Page No.**	**Reps/Time**	
1	Barbell Rollouts	110	8 to 10	
2	Saxon Side Bends	112	8 to 10 on each side	
3	Hanging Leg Raises	114	8 to 10	
4	Full-Contact Twists	122	6 to 8 on each side	
5	Dead Lifts	128	6 to 10	

Perform exercises as a circuit (one exercise after the other); rest 1 minute and then repeat entire circuit once or twice.

DAY 2			FOCUS: CORE STRENGTH AND POWER	
No.	**Exercise**	**Page No.**	**Reps/Time**	
1	Medicine Ball Kneeling Throw	94	6 to 10	
2	Swiss Ball Lower Body Rotations	84	6 to 8 on each side	
3	Medicine Ball Woodchopper	96	6 to 10	
4	V-Up	52	8 to 10	
5	Good Mornings	132	6 to 8	

Perform exercises as a circuit (one exercise after the other); rest 1 minute and then repeat entire circuit once or twice.

DAY 3			FOCUS: CORE STABILITY AND STRENGTH	
No.	**Exercise**	**Page No.**	**Reps/Time**	
1	Slow Sit-Up	56	10 to 12	
2	Swiss Ball Reverse Crunch	70	8 to 10	
3	Swiss Ball Lower Body Rotations	84	6 to 8 on each side	
4	Lateral Bridge	58	6 to 10 on each side	
5	Suitcase Dead Lifts	134	6 to 8 on each side	

Perform exercises as a circuit (one exercise after the other); rest 1 minute and then repeat entire circuit once or twice.

14-Day Ab Sculpting Workout #1: Weeks 3 & 4

SPECIAL INSTRUCTIONS FOR WEEKS 3 & 4

- Perform three ab workouts each week. Incorporate two to three total-body strength workouts and two to three days of interval cardio in your program.
- Start with a general warm-up and then proceed to the Ab Warm-Ups (pages 26 to 43) before beginning these workouts.
- On Day 2 add enough resistence to the exercises so that your muscles are fatiguing during the last few reps, but not enough weight to destroy your form. (See page 142).
- Perform exercises as supersets.

DAY 1			FOCUS: CORE STABILITY AND STRENGTH
No.	Exercise	Page No.	Reps/Time
1	Barbell Rollouts	110	8 to 10
2	Saxon Side Bends	112	8 to 10 on each side

Perform these two exercises as a circuit; rest 1 minute and then repeat circuit once or twice.

1	Hanging Leg Raises	114	8 to 10
2	Full Contact Twists	122	6 to 8 on each side

Perform these two exercises as a circuit; rest 1 minute and then repeat circuit once or twice.

DAY 2			FOCUS: CORE STABILITY AND ROTATIONAL POWER
No.	Exercise	Page No.	Reps/Time
1	Medicine Ball Kneeling Throw	94	4 to 6
2	Swiss Ball Lower Body Rotations	84	6 to 8 on each side

Perform these two exercises as a circuit; rest 1 minute and then repeat circuit once or twice.

1	Medicine Ball Woodchopper	96	4 to 6
2	Good Mornings	132	6 to 8

Perform these two exercises as a circuit; rest 1 minute and then repeat circuit once or twice.

DAY 3			FOCUS: CORE STABILITY AND STRENGTH
No.	Exercise	Page No.	Reps/Time
1	Slow Sit-Up	56	10 to 12
2	Swiss Ball Reverse Crunch	70	8 to 10

Perform these two exercises as a circuit; rest 1 minute and then repeat circuit once or twice.

1	Swiss Ball Lower Body Rotations	84	6 to 8 on each side
2	Lateral Bridge	58	6 to 10 on each side

Perform these two exercises as a circuit; rest 1 minute and then repeat circuit once or twice.

1	Suitcase Dead Lifts	134	6 to 8 on each side

Complete two to three sets; rest 1 minute between sets

14-Day Ab Sculpting Workout #1: Weeks 5 & 6

SPECIAL INSTRUCTIONS FOR WEEKS 5 & 6

- Perform three ab workouts each week. Incorporate two to three total-body strength workouts and two to three days of interval cardio in your program.
- Start with a general warm-up and then proceed to the Ab Warm-Ups (pages 26 to 43) before beginning these workouts.
- Add enough resistence to these exercises so that your muscles are fatiguing during the last few reps, but not enough weight to destroy your form. (See page 142).

DAY 1			FOCUS: STRENGTH AND EXPLOSIVE POWER
No.	Exercise	Page No.	Reps/Time
1	Knee-In	60	4 to 7
2	Swiss Ball Oblique Crunch	72	4 to 7
3	Medicine Ball Kneeling Throw	94	4 to 7
4	Supermans	126	4 to 7

Perform exercises as a circuit; rest 1 minute and then repeat entire circuit once or twice.

DAY 2			FOCUS: ROTATIONAL POWER
No.	Exercise	Page No.	Reps/Time
1	Medicine Ball Woodchopper	96	4 to 7
2	Swiss Ball Lower Body Rotations	84	4 to 7
3	Vacuum	46	4 to 7

Perform exercises as a circuit; rest 1 minute and then repeat entire circuit once or twice.

DAY 3			FOCUS: CORE STABILITY
No.	Exercise	Page No.	Reps/Time
1	Crunch with Lateral Flexion	50	10 to 15
2	Oblique V-Up	54	10 to 15
3	Overhead Squats	130	10 to 15

Perform exercises as a circuit; rest 1 minute and then repeat entire circuit once or twice.